1395

W9-BTC-339

History, Trends, and Politics of Nursing

Vern L. Bullough, R.N., Ph.D.
Dean
Natural and Social Sciences
State University College at Buffalo
Buffalo, New York

Bonnie Bullough, R.N., Ph.D.
Dean
School of Nursing
State University of New York at Buffalo
Buffalo, New York

APPLETON-CENTURY-CROFTS/Norwalk, Connecticut

0-8385-3775-8

Notice: The authors and publisher of this volume have taken care that the information and recommendations contained herein are accurate and compatible with the standards generally accepted at the time of publication.

84 85 86 87 88 / 10 9 8 7 6 5 4 3 2 1

Prentice-Hall International, Inc., London
Prentice-Hall of Australia, Pty. Ltd., Sydney
Prentice-Hall Canada, Inc.
Prentice-Hall of India Private Limited, New Delhi
Prentice-Hall of Japan, Inc., Tokyo
Prentice-Hall of Southeast Asia (Pte.) Ltd., Singapore
Whitehall Books Ltd., Wellington, New Zealand
Editora Prentice-Hall do Brasil Ltda., Rio de Janeiro

Library of Congress Cataloging in Publication Data

Bullough, Vern L.
   History, trends, and politics of nursing.
   Includes bibliographical references and index.
   1. Nursing—History. 2. Nursing—Social aspects.
3. Nursing—Political aspects. I. Bullough, Bonnie.
II. Title. [DNLM: 1. Nursing—Trends. 2. History
of nursing. WY 11.1 B938h]
RT31.B83   1984   610.73   83-25874
ISBN 0-8385-3775-8

Design: Lynn M. Luchetti

PRINTED IN THE UNITED STATES OF AMERICA

Contents

Preface

Earlier generations of nurses studied nursing history in order to locate nursing within a larger framework and to examine current trends in nursing. In the 1960s and 1970s nursing history went through a period of neglect, only to be defined as important again in the 1980s. Nowhere is this new importance more evident than in the recently-recommended criteria for accreditation of nursing programs by the National League for Nursing, calling for analysis of the historical, legal, political, social and ethical aspects of nursing to be included in the curriculum. Hopefully, this book will do just that, even though it was completed before the NLN criteria appeared. Instead, our analysis of what should be taught in nursing fortuitously agreed with what the NLN also saw as a perceived need.

The book is not a definitive text on any of the subjects mentioned above. Rather, it is an overview, distilling what we have written elsewhere about history, law, politics, ethics and social issues. Hopefully, it will whet the appetite of both students and non-students, encouraging them to read more deeply into the areas we have examined. To this end, we have included references and a guide for further reading. Simply studying the issues raised in the book, however, is not enough. We strongly believe that nurses themselves can be agents of change rather than simply being pushed along by the currents of time. To act as change agents, however, nurses need a clear idea of where nursing has been and what the options are for the future. It is also important to become active in groups and organizations bringing about change. We hope this book will be helpful in this respect as well.

Special thanks to Judy Stolzman, Debra Heisler, and Suzanne Macie-jewski, who typed the final manuscript. Charles Bollinger, Senior Editor, and Douglas Gall, Production Editor, also deserve thanks for their support and encouragement.

Introduction

One of the things that nursing teaches us is that the major key to understanding patient problems is an adequate patient history. What is true of a patient is true for a profession and even for a society. That is why we have the discipline of history. Issues in nursing did not suddenly appear—they have a history—and without examining that history, we cannot understand either where nursing is coming from or where it is going. Just as the patient's history gives us certain clues as to diagnosis and treatment, so does the history of a profession. Such a history, however, only serves as a starting point, as a kind of guide, and ultimate diagnosis is dependent on a number of other tests and procedures. In dealing with larger groups of people, those tests and procedures come from the fields of sociology and political science, and so we periodically stop to use tools from those fields along with history to evaluate where we are. Just as it is necessary to offer some kind of treatment or regimen to the patient, so it is necessary to make some decisions about the profession. These decisions can be meaningful. The paths of development that nursing might follow are not inevitable but are dependent on what we do and what we want. We have several options open to us, and the options we choose at this point open up different sets of options down the road. Today's options are not tomorrow's because options change with time. Similarly, our options are different from those of our predecessors, and our choices must, perforce, be different. Still, all too often, basic problems recur; they just reappear in different forms. Thus, we have to keep on resolving the same issues as they appear in different guises. History is particularly important because it gives us insights about current problems and helps us to identify recurrent problems.

NURSING IDENTITY: AN ANCIENT AND RECURRING PROBLEM

Although nursing, as we know it, is primarily a late nineteenth-century development, it has always been around, and yet it was not always clearly identified as an "occupation" separate from medicine. One of the major problems in looking at the history of nursing is distinguishing between nursing and medicine. This problem is complicated by the fact that health care today is hierarchically organized under the dominance of physicians who have tended to claim all past health care developments as their own.

In spite of such claims, it is possible to distinguish a nursing role, even in the prehistoric period. We know, for example, from skeletal evidence as well as later written records, that people in the past who were ill or wounded or otherwise incapacitated and unable to care for themselves somehow survived. This implies that someone took care of them, feeding them, cleaning them, giving them emotional support. In this sense, the nurse predates the physician, and it could be argued that only after observing and caring for the ill and incapacitated for long periods did anyone acquire enough expertise to intervene. Intervention itself did not distinguish the nurse from the physician. Rather, the basic difference was the interrelationship of the physician with the priest or shaman. Often they were the same person since the healing process, in spite of one's experience in patient care, is not always predictable. Ancient people knew this, and although they recognized that such things as poisons, wounds, burns, and falls would affect their health, or even kill them, and that cold, heat, too much sun, overstraining, or overeating might cause some minor discomfort or ailment, different people recovered or failed to recover at different rates. This led to the belief that death and suffering included a supernatural or magical component that had to be dealt with and gave the physician-shaman-priest greater power than the more empirically trained nurses, establishing his position at the top of the health hierarchy.

It was this priestly association that enabled the physician to emerge as a clearly defined historical figure much earlier than the nurse, since writing was closely associated with the clerical class. Other than his authority position, however, the physician still did many of the tasks that nurses did. In fact, until almost the twentieth century, the physician was supposed to stay with his patient until various crises had been overcome or passed through. This meant that the physician's services were restricted to the wealthy and powerful while the poor were, as always, dependent on lesser status figures such as nurses or midwives.

Historically, the line between the two, medicine and nursing, has gone through several changes. Although family members often served as nurses, there has always existed the need for more sophisticated care. In the Hippocratic corpus, that is the writing prevalent in the Greek world of the third century B.C. and which is attributed to Hippocrates of Cos, there are references to assistants to the physician who were delegated to observe the patient. These might well have been physicians in training (Hippocrates, 1967). In the times of Roman supremacy, the Romans found need for a more sophisticated nursing system to support their armies, who often found themselves far away from home. The solution was the forerunner of the hospital system, originally a series of tents arranged on a kind of corridor system. Eventually, tents gave way to buildings that became permanent convalescent camps. These hospitals contained wards, recreation areas, baths, pharmacies, rooms for attendants, and even luxury rooms for officials taking a cure. Although there were physicians attached to each Roman legion, the key unit was the hospital. A description exists in the writings of Vegetius, who emphasized the military discipline maintained in them. The man who nursed his comrades-in-arms was called a *contubernalis*—literally a tent companion. These were supplemented by others known simply as attendants or adjutants. There were also civilian hospitals, and every large estate had a *valetudinarium*, or hospital, which was to be supervised by the bailiff or official in charge of the estate (Vegetius, 1944).

In the early medieval period, a further change took place in these hospitals, one that had great influence on nursing, namely, the appearance of a religious commitment as part of the nursing profession. Since the Christian church expressed great concern for the poor, the sick, and the afflicted, it was natural that people who dealt with them be regarded as having a special calling. The result was the development of the *xendochium*, a kind of hospital designed to care for those who could not or would not be cared for in their own homes. Included in this group were the traveler or pilgrim, the poor and the destitute, the orphan and abandoned children, the elderly, and the plague-stricken. Both men and women worked in these institutions. Their primary function was to take care of the needs of the inmates, physical as well as emotional. This "Christianizing" of the nurse's calling helped further to distinguish nursing from medicine. Religion forced nurses then, and even now, to make a commitment, with money, family, and personal freedom all being sacrificed. The physician was not part of the movement. Instead, medicine tended to emphasize knowledge and ability rather than commitment. Religious commitment in nursing was further strengthened with the appearance and growth of monasticism in the fourth and fifth centuries in the West. The care of the sick fell increasingly to those men and women who chose the religious life, assisted by the patients themselves. We have an eleventh-century description of a large hospital in Constantinople by Anna Comnena, the daughter of the Emperor Alexius. She reported that in the hospital, patients could be seen

> . . . walking along, sometimes blind, sometimes lame, sometimes having some other ill, and seeing it, you would say it was Solomon's Porch filled with men incapacitated in their limbs. I, myself, have seen an old woman waited on by a young one, and a blind man led by a seeing man, and a footless man using the feet not of himself, but of others, and a handless man led by the hands of other men, and children nursed by strange mothers, and paralytics served by able-bodied mortals. So the number of those who were supported was double, some being served and some servers. Thus, Alexius gave attendants to each incapacitated man. (Comnena, 1928)

As the West itself began to send out crusading armies, the need for effective care of the sick and wounded again became acute. Out of this need came the nursing orders, including the Knights of St. John (Hospitallers), and the Knights Templar. The nurses in these orders were required to visit the sick in their hospitals, both mornings and evenings. The bed linens and other supplies were under the nurse's charge, and the assistants under him washed the feet of the sick, changed their linen, fed the weak, and, in general, helped the sick. In the growing cities of the West, the monastic hospitals also grew and spread. Just how much contact the patients in such hospitals had with physicians is debatable. In retrospect, it seems as if nursing existed almost independently of medicine.

With the appearance of Protestantism in the sixteenth century, the hospital movement in much of Europe lost ground. This was because the Protestants abolished the religious orders, and without them, hospitals apparently could not function. When people complained about the lack of institutions for the ill, as they did in England, some hospitals made a reappearance, but the attendants in them were trained at a much lower level than in the medieval ones and generally lacked the religious commitment. Traditional hospitals continued to exist in Catholic countries, and so most of the early hospitals established in the United States and Canada were established in those areas where there were Catholic communities.

Medicine coped with the loss of the existing nursing care by ignoring large segments of the population or leaving them to other practitioners, such as apothecaries or midwives, or simply to women who had earned a reputation as healers. Still, the cost to medicine of the loss of effective nursing was high. Physicians could not specialize because they had to take every patient who could afford their fees. Since they had to spend long hours with their patients, seeing them through their individual crises and following them closely, the number of patients a physician could have was severely limited. Patients were also neglected, particularly in the rapidly growing cities where the citizens lacked the family support system that existed in the small towns and villages. Many simply had no place to go when they were ill. Out of this came agitation for a reinvigoration of nursing, a movement that climaxed in the efforts of Florence Nightingale to establish a different kind of nurse. With the Nightingale nurse as the foundation, the hospitals could expand very rapidly, permitting physicians to delegate much of their traditional overseeing of patient care to nurses. In this phase of nursing, however, almost everything that came to be defined as nursing had been done previously either by the physician or the patient's family.

NURSES VERSUS PHYSICIANS

At first, nurses did not take temperatures. Then they were allowed to take temperatures but not blood pressures, and then blood pressures but not something else. Each extension of the nurse's role was at the expense of the physicians (from some viewpoints), and from taking over these functions, a new nurse's role began to emerge. This role has continued to change as conditions have changed, but usually modern nursing has been defined in terms of medicine. This fact has often antagonized nurses who have sought various ways of asserting independence from medicine. Although medicine is equally dependent on nursing, the status differences favor physicians, and they have paid much less attention to what nurses do than nurses pay to what they do.

One way of coping has been to emphasize a nursing assessment separate and distinct from a medical diagnosis. The nursing assessment or diagnosis focuses more on the patient's needs, giving more account to the psychosocial factors of illness than a medical diagnosis, but it cannot ignore the physiological aspects of illness. Some state laws were written to mark this nursing independence from medicine, but courts generally have been unable to distinguish between a nursing assessment and a medical diagnosis, except to indicate that one might be performed by a nurse and the other by a physician. In a sense, some of the play on words is an effort to avoid medicine jumping on nursing, and by adopting the term nursing assessment, nurses are doing what psychologists did a few years ago when they ran into trouble with the use of the term therapy (a term the physicians claimed for themselves). To avoid conflict, the psychologists indicated that they were merely counseling the patient, but gradually it soon became apparent that there was little difference between counseling and therapy, and today the two terms are often used interchangeably by the psychologist. Nursing has not yet been as successful, although it often has adopted different terms than those used by the physician, using, for example, maternal and child health instead of obstetrics and pediatrics. Thus we can insist we are not following a medical model, but a nursing one.

Nurses also adopted coping mechanisms on the floors to assert their own integrity, even though they knew the hospital was dominated by physicians. One coping mechanism was the doctor-nurse game, a variant of the man-woman game in which women, while nominally accepting male "dominance," indirectly assert their own independence. The game is based on the assumption that all patient care decisions are made by physicians, which generally is not true because physicians are not present when most care is given. When game-playing nurses make decisions, they handle the situation by invoking the name of the doctor to the patient and pretending to the doctors that their (the nurses') ideas were the doctors'.

The conflict between nursing and medicine is also basic to some internal conflicts in nursing itself. To oversimplify, this conflict is between those nurses who want to work closely with physicians and incorporate technical medical skills in their role and those nurses who seek to distance themselves from medicine and carve out an independent nursing role focused on the social-psychological aspects of patient care. At the specialty level, the nurses with medical elements in their role include the nurse practitioners, nurse midwives, nurse anesthetists, and critical care nurses, whereas the clinical specialists are the more psychologically oriented group. The dominant mood of the profession in recent decades probably favors the independent social-psychological focus. Consequently, nursing history is full of examples of groups of nurses who have set up their own organizations and even their own training centers because organized and official nursing had refused to recognize what they did as proper nursing. At the bedside level, this conflict is represented by an effort on the part of certain groups to make a distinction between care and cure. These groups regard the care nurse as having a higher status than the one who "simply does the required tasks" necessary for curing. In retrospect, one of the motivations behind this dichotomy was an effort to emphasize the social-psychological skills of the baccalaureate-trained nurse as against the more technically trained associate and training school graduate, but it was also an effort to carve out certain areas of health care from the physician and claim nurse expertise. This is an issue on which nurses still disagree, but it is an example of where history might throw some light. This conflict is discussed in more depth in later chapters.

REFERENCES

For general reading:
Bullough, V.L. & Bullough, B. *The care of the sick: The emergence of modern nursing.* New York: Neale Watson, Prodist, 1978.

Comnena, A. *Alexiad* Bk. XV, 7. E.A.S. Dawes (Trans.). London: Kegan Paul, Trench Trubner, 1928.
Hippocrates, Decorum, XVII. In *Hippocrates* Vol. II, W.H.S. Jones and E.T. Withington (Eds. and Trans.). London: William Heinemann, 1967.
Vegetius. *Military institutions of the romans,* III, 2. John Clark (Ed. and Trans.). Harrisburg, Pa.: Military Service Publishing, 1944.

Section I
NURSES AS WOMEN

CHAPTER 1

The Subordinate Sex

If a dominant theme of nursing politics has been the struggle for identity vis-à-vis physicians, it has been complicated by the fact that modern nursing has been regarded as a woman's profession. This was not the case in all historical periods. While it is true that throughout the ages most sick people were cared for in their homes by unpaid relatives, and most of these caretakers were women, the early nurses were men. Most of the battlefield nursing was done by men. The early monastic orders included both monks and nuns. By the late Middle Ages, that balance shifted toward women, and nursing sisters came to dominate the field. Nursing in the Protestant countries in the pre-Nightingale era was done by both sexes, with more women than men in the field. Nightingale further stamped the profession as a female occupation. Today, 1 out of every 44 women is a nurse, and although men have been entering the profession in increased numbers in the last decade, women remain the dominant and influential voice.

Some of the Nightingale influence in the direction of making nursing so female-oriented was personal, but some of it had to do with nineteenth century societal norms. It is difficult for men and women of today to realize how circumscribed a woman's life was in the past. Mary Wollstonecraft (1759–1797), whose *Vindication of the Rights of Woman* (1792) is a kind of manifesto for future generations of women, made a passionate plea for the education of women.

> Men complain, and with reason, of the follies and caprices of our sex, when they do not keenly satirize our headstrong passions and groveling vices. Behold, I should answer the natural effect of ignorance! The mind will ever be unstable that has only prejudices to

rest on, and the current will run with destructive fury when there are no barriers to break its force. Women are told from their infancy, and taught by the examples of their mothers, that a little knowledge of human weakness, justly termed cunning, softness of temper, outward obedience, and a scrupulous attention to a puerile kind of propriety, will obtain for them the protection of man; and should they be beautiful, everything else is needless, for at least twenty years of their lives. (Woolstonecraft, 1929)

Women's every action was under the legal control of a male, whether father, brother, husband, or son, and women's activities were carefully circumscribed both by law and by tradition. There were, however, class distinctions; upper-class women had somewhat more freedom than middle-class women. There was also a real distinction between middle-class and working-class women, in that working-class women were permitted to seek employment outside the home if they could, and in the industrial revolution of the eighteenth and nineteenth centuries, large numbers of women did find employment in the factories, particularly in the textile factories. In 1730 Daniel Defoe, best known for his novel *Robinson Crusoe*, explained the importance of female employment in *A Plan of the English Commerce*. He pointed out that a

. . . poor labouring Man that goes abroad to his Day Work, and Husbandry, Hedging, Ditching, Threshing, Carting, etc. and brings home his Week's Wages, suppose at eight Pence to twelve Pence a Day, or in some Counties less; if he has a Wife and three or four Children to feed, and who get little or nothing for themselves, must fare hard, and live poorly; 'tis easy to suppose it must be so. But if this Man's Wife and Children can at the same Time get Employment . . . . This alters the Case extremely, the Family feels it, they all feed better, are cloth'd warmer, and do not so easily nor so often fall into Misery or Distress. (Defoe, 1730)

Because factories gave women an opportunity to move outside the home and ultimately led to a shift in their outlook, they broke down some of the confinement to which women had been subject. There was, however, considerable ambivalence about this development both by women and by men. Many argued that the employment of women was an "inversion of the order of nature and of Providence— a return to a state of barbarism in which the woman does the work, while the man looks idly on." (Defoe, 1730) Increasingly, it was the single woman, not the married woman, who worked in the factory, and such a discrimination was probably accepted by a married woman on the grounds that her earnings usually did not make up for the loss to the family resulting from the nonperformance of other domestic duties. The nineteenth century also tended to put rigid restrictions on what a woman could or could not do in the factory. Certain tasks, such as mining, ultimately came to be declared unsuitable for women because they were too heavy or required working in confined spaces that were not conducive to the best of moral behavior. Still, in a crisis, a woman of the working classes, married or unmarried, could work outside the home. No such activity was permitted to the middle-class woman who found outlets for her energies more and more restricted. Margaretta Greg, writing in 1853, complained that a lady must be a mere lady and nothing else:

> She must not work for profit, or engage in any occupation that money can command, lest she invade the rights of the working classes, who live by their labour. Men in want of employment have pressed their way into nearly all the shopping and retail businesses that in my early years were managed in whole, or in part, by women. The conventional barrier that pronounced it ungenteel to be behind a counter, or serving the public in any mercantile capacity, is greatly extended. The same in household economy. Servants must be up to their offices, which is very well; but ladies, dismissed from the dairy, the confectionery, the store room, the still room, the poultry yard, the kitchen garden, and the orchard have hardly yet found themselves a sphere equally useful and important to the pursuits of trade and arts to which to apply their too abundant leisure. (Greg, in Pinchbeck, 1969)

It was from the educated middle-class women who became more and more unhappy with their confined role in society that the demands for female emancipation began to appear. Florence Nightingale, although more well-to-do than some of her American counterparts, came from this group. Tied in with the lack of economic opportunities was the model of gentility that proper women were to attain. A woman was expected to be a model of self control, to deny or attenuate sexual attraction as the mode of relation between the sexes, and to favor discreet withdrawal and even retreat in the face of vulgarity. It was absolutely essential that women in their appearance exhibit a meticulous personal daintiness, have an absence of "violent" muscularity in any of their gestures, and their clothes and hairdress were to display an unfunctional fragility. This meant that even in her "creative" activities there were limits to which a woman could channel her energies. Music was a favorite pastime for many because it could show their femininity at its best, but the restrictions in this field emphasize the restrictions in other fields since so many musical activities were unladylike. If a girl played a flute or a horn, she had to purse her lips, a very unladylike gesture; the brass instruments had the added difficulty of requiring visceral support for tone quality, which meant they were even more unladylike. The cello required a girl to spread her legs; if she played a violin, she had to twist her upper torso and strain her neck in an unnatural way. The clothes of the time added to the difficulties of playing and remaining ladylike. In fact, about the only instrument a proper girl could play was a keyboard one; the harpsichord, clavichord, or pianoforte allowed the girl to sit properly before the keyboard, arrange her clothes neatly, put a polite smile on her face, keep her feet demurely together, strike the key lightly with no unseemly vehemence, and act gentle and genteel, an outward symbol of her family's ability to pay for her education and her decorativeness. When she played, a woman was not to perform like a professional but play adequately, a symbol of the fact that she did not have to work and did not have to chase after men.

Inevitably, the life of the proper woman came to be filled with a kind of genteel idleness in which she tried to fill her time with a number of trivial diversions superficially related to the fine arts known as "accomplishments": fancy needlework and embroidery; framing pictures in shellwork; embellishing cabinets with a tracery of seaweed, filigree, and varnish work; working with chenille, crepe, ribbon, or netting; making artificial flowers of wax or fabric; cutting out paper ornaments; drawing or painting slightly; and playing the piano adequately. When anything untoward appeared, the lady was either to withdraw or, if this were impossible, to faint. There were even ways to faint elegantly:

> The eyes grow dim, and almost closed; the jaw fallen; the head hung down; as if too heavy to be supported by the neck. A general inertia prevails. The voice trembling, the utterance through the nose; every sentence accompanied with a groan; the hand shaking, and the knees tottering under the body. Fainting eventually produces a sudden relaxation of all that holds the human frame together, every sinew and ligament unstrung. The colour flies from the vermilion cheek; the sparkling eye grows dim. Down the body drops, as helpless, and as senseless, as a mass of clay, to which, by its colour and appearance it seems hastening to resolve itself. (Defoe, 1782)

Woman's task was to be a homemaker and mother, and because she was weak, she had to be safeguarded at all costs from the corrupting effects of the man-made world. The burden put on women by such attitudes was one that many did not want and could not bear, but about the only outlet for their discontent was church work, or literary pursuits, such as Jane Austen and the Brontë sisters managed to do. Religion, in a sense, became justification for what many women wanted to do and could not do, and inevitably, even woman's suffrage became a movement to raise the standards of morality by allowing the purer and finer species, the women, to vote. Women were taught to think of themselves as a special class, and having become conscious of their unique sexual identity, they were forced to play their role. Denied liberty, they sought power, and not infrequently, the easiest way to gain power was through their children. Motherhood came to be elevated to a kind of mystique which Freud made into a kind of pseudoscientific basis of existence. Although the nineteenth-century concept of women (some would call it Victorian) as wan, ethereal, spiritualized creatures bore little relation to the real world where women operated machines, worked the fields, hand-washed clothing, toiled over great kitchen stoves, it was endorsed by science and religion. Fashion assisted materially by keeping women in bustles and hoops, corsets and trailing skirts, and other items of clothing in which they remained encased throughout much of the period. The ideal waist came to be the span of a man's two hands, and since few women could achieve this naturally, they did so by tight lacing. Feminine delicacy, which was so admired, was at least in part due to constricting corsets rather than visible evidence of the superior sensibilities, the "finer clay" of which women were made. Women who were not delicate by nature became so by design. Most women came to believe in their own special genius, and those who did not conform were usually ostracized. The world came to be made up of good girls and bad girls. The bad girls represented sexuality, and the good girls represented purity of mind and spirit, unclouded by the shadow of any gross or vulgar thought.

It was on this background that secular nursing appeared. Although it entailed contact with the real world of the sick and the wounded, and thereby was not suited for a lady, in another sense, it fit the supportive, caring, nurturing role of the proper woman. It also had a religious connotation. In fact, throughout the first part of the nineteenth century, a number of health care reformers had tried to establish various kinds of religious orders devoted to nursing, tracing the authority for these back to the Deaconess movement active in the very early Christian church. Particularly influential in Protestant countries were the nursing movements started by Pastor Theodore Fliedner (1800–1864) in Kaiserswerth, now a part of West Germany, and Elizabeth Fry (1780–1845) in England. The religious impetus behind these reforms is all-important because it was through a religious calling that women in Western culture traditionally have been able to escape some of the limitations put on them. It was in the name of religion, for example, that women such as St. Catherine of Siena or St. Theresa could play a central role in European history, and it was in the name of a religious commitment that Florence Nightingale was able to become a nurse.

Nightingale (1820–1910) came from the well-to-do middle classes where women had the most limitations. She had greater freedom than most girls of her class, however, since her father was determined that she and her sister (Parthenope) would be well educated, and instead of hiring a governess, he took the education of his daughters upon himself. Under his direction, they learned Greek, Latin, German, French, Italian, history, and philosophy, and through special tutors, they learned enough music and drawing to be regarded as cultivated women. In fact, Florence was one of the best-educated women in Europe in her time, although she herself felt her weakness was mathematics. Women in Florence's social class were supposed to devote themselves to society, entertainment, and similar pursuits, but the young Nightingale had other ideas, and although we know she was attractive and enjoyed dancing, parties, and boys, she wanted to be her own mistress.

Religion provided the way, and she recorded that God spoke to her and called her to His service. The date was February 7, 1837, and she was not yet 17. Later, she underwent three similar experiences. The immediate problem, however, was her mother, who wanted her to get married and settle down, something that Florence refused to do. Girls of her class, however, did not openly oppose their mothers, at least not directly, and so for several years, she and her mother fought a ladylike battle over what Florence was going to do.

Part of the difficulty was that she did not know what she wanted to do with her life, and it was only in 1844 after considerable thought and study, that she decided that her vocation lay among the sick. She began to gain experience by nursing relatives, and while doing this, she made a rather startling discovery that just being a woman did not guarantee being a good nurse. She soon realized that tenderness, sympathy, goodness, and patience were good qualities for a nurse to have, but without knowledge and skill, in other words, training, the would-be nurse could do little. To receive such training, she tried to persuade her family to allow her to learn nursing at a nearby infirmary, but this caused her mother to have hysterics, and Nightingale, herself, took to her bed, an acceptable feminine way of coping in the nineteenth century. Unable to learn nursing through first-hand experience, she began to read hospital and sanitary reports, books on what we now call public health, and the yearbook of the Kaiserwerth Institutions founded by Pastor Fliedner. Through her reading, she gained a greater understanding of hospitals and the care of the sick than almost any of her contemporaries, male or female.

The more book knowledge she gained, the more she felt the need for some practicum. Her mother (her father was now dead) continued to oppose her, and from 1844 to 1851, mother and daughter engaged in a struggle of wills until finally, in spite of opposition from her family, she got up enough courage to visit Kaiserwerth in 1851. After her return from Kaiserwerth, she was determined to go to Paris to study further with the Sisters of Charity. The opposition of her mother and sister to this trip was so violent that Florence, for a time, thought her going would endanger her sister's life. Still, she perservered. She had only been in Paris a short time before being requested to come home to take care of her dying grandmother. Ever the dutiful daughter, she returned. It should be added that on both these expeditions, she was properly chaperoned.

Shortly after her grandmother died in 1853, the Institution for the Care of Sick Gentlewomen in Distressed Circumstances (institutional names at that time were long and self-explanatory) found itself in difficulty, and the women in charge, friends of Florence's mother and of the proper social class, asked Nightingale to take over the superintendency. In spite of familial opposition, Florence agreed, and surprisingly once the decision was made, her mother and sister accepted the idea. Perhaps one reason they did was that they had begun to accept the fact that Florence was not going to marry; they could also console themselves that the women who ran the home were of the proper social class, and the patients themselves came from their own class. Once in charge, Nightingale put ideas and concepts into effect that she had been thinking about for some time: bells were installed for patients to ring, lifts were built to bring food to the floors so that the attendants would not have to leave their wards, and all religious requirements for admission were abolished. The committee had balked at this last change, but Nightingale, determined to have her way, carried the day. Nursing care was so improved that her patients were reported to have worshipped her. She was still not satisfied, however, and one of the greatest deficiencies she noted was the lack of trained nurses. Simply raising the standards of nursing in one institution was not enough; what was needed was an upgrading of nursing training. In order to begin to solve this problem, she entered negotiations to become superintendent of nurses at the newly reorganized and rebuilt King's College Hospital in London, but before negotiations proceeded very far, the Crimean War broke out, and the life of Florence Nightingale and the nature of nursing changed.

The Crimean War, which started with England and France declaring war on Russia in March 1854 and sending their armies off to the Crimea, was a history of blunders and stupidities. No real preparation had been made for supplying the army in the Crimea. In the first battles, there were no bandages, splints, chloroform, or other drugs; the wounded lay on the ground or in straw mixed with manure in the farm yards; amputations were performed without anesthetics with the victims sitting or lying on tubs or on old doors, and surgeons caught without candles or lamps did much of their work by moonlight. Cholera created havoc. As the casualties rose, the Turkish government (ally of the English and the French) turned over to the British the enormous barracks at Scutari, across the straits from Constantinople. No hospital equipment was put in the barracks, which were bare, filthy, and dilapidated, but the wounded and sick were sent there anyway. They were put on the floor and wrapped in blankets saturated with blood; no food was given to them because there was no kitchen; no one could attend to their wounds because there was a shortage of surgeons; many of the wounded lay without even a drink of water all night because there were no cups or buckets to bring water.

Such incompetence and neglect was not particularly unusual in wartime in the past, but the Crimean War was different because it marked the first appearance of war correspondents. It was the beginning of circulation battles among newspapers for the increasingly literate masses, and the result was a real public awareness of the tragedies affecting the British army. The reporters, primarily William Howard Russell of the *London Times,* described in great detail the lack of care for the wounded and the horrible suffering they had to undergo. Newspaper editorials soon thundered, demanding to know why the sick lacked adequate care. British nursing service was compared to the French nursing service under the care of the Sisters of Charity, and criticism of the government mounted to such a level that there was a danger it could be voted out of office.

In this situation, Secretary of War Sidney Herbert, an old friend of Florence Nightingale who was knowledgeable about what she was doing, wrote to her on October 15, 1854 asking her to gather together a group of nurses and lead them to Scutari. Even before hearing from Herbert, Nightingale had begun arrangements to sail to Constantinople with a group of nurses, and her letter offering her services and Herbert's requesting them apparently crossed in the mail. Nightingale acted quickly, and a departure date was set for

October 21, which left her less than a week to recruit her nurses, find equipment and uniforms, and arrange transportation.

The announcement of her appointment caused a sensation, for she was the first woman ever to serve in such a capacity. Her mother and sister forgot their previous opposition to her plans, and were, to put it simply, ecstatic. Although we regard Nightingale as the founder of secular nursing, most of the nurses who accompanied her to Crimea were from religious orders, either Catholic or Protestant. There were only 14 secular nurses among the 38 nurses who accompanied her.

From the beginning, there was considerable dissension among the different contingents of nurses because of Nightingale's dictatorial methods. Since no would-be rival had her political backing, she remained in more-or-less absolute control. Some indication of her backing was the fact that she was given a special fund raised by the readers of the *London Times* to spend as she would. She also had the personal support of Queen Victoria.

When the women arrived in Scutari, they found that the chaos and confusion pictured by the newspapers had not been exaggerated. Many officers told Nightingale she would "spoil the brutes" if she took over the responsibility for the sick and wounded since they were only "animals," "blackguards," or "scum." Medical authorities were outraged by what they considered her unreasonable demands for clean bedding, hot soup, hospital clothing, or other such "preposterous luxuries." To make matters even worse, she was a woman, and the surgeons at Scutari had decided that what they least needed was a society lady and a pack of female nurses. At first, they either ignored her or adopted an attitude of outward submission in deference to her powerful political backing and then proceeded to hamstring her whenever or however they could. Nightingale soon realized what was going on, and rather than confront them, she reverted to a traditional female role, sitting back and waiting for the males to request her assistance. She chose, however, to sit in sight of everyone, sorting linens or provisions and doing other busy work, and gave strict orders for her nurses to leave the patients alone. This tactic irritated many of her nurses who wanted to alleviate the suffering around them, but Nightingale would not tolerate opposition. Nurses were there, she said, to assist the surgeon, not to run the hospital.

Her first entry into the hospital was through the kitchen, the place where the medical men least resented her influence, probably because they regarded it as traditional woman's work. At Scutari, before her arrival, the only utensils for cooking had been some 13 Turkish kettles holding 450 pints each. Meat was issued by wards, and each ward steward tossed his ration into the pot. Since there were no stirring spoons available, meat that landed on the bottom was well cooked, while that which went in last was hardly cooked at all. Each ward steward put a distinguishing mark on the ward's meat—a red rag, an old nail, surgical scissors, or a piece of uniform—so they could identify what was theirs. All the meat was removed together and theoretically taken to the patient, but many received no food at all. Once the meat had been removed from the kettle, tea was made in the same kettle, and since water was in short supply, the kettles were not even washed. Nightingale, at first, began to cook extras from her own supplies and with her own equipment, the surgeons allowing her to give these meals to certain patients. Within a week, her kitchen had become what we would now call a diet kitchen. Soon after this, she took over all cooking, and for five months, she was the only source of food for the hospitals.

On November 9, the whole hospital opened up to her as a result of the almost total collapse of the British army in the Crimea from exposure, scurvy, starvation, dysentery, and Russian defensive action. As winter set in, the hospital at Scutari was overrun with patients; in fact, more soldiers were in the hospital than at the front. In desperation, the doctors were forced to turn to Nightingale and her nurses— in fact, to anyone who was willing to help. The women responded to the tragic situation with speed and determination. Some indication of the level care had reached was the fact that more than 1,000 men suffered from acute diarrhea when the nurses were allowed on the wards, but there were only 20 chamber pots in the whole hospital. Moreover, the privies were useless, so overflowing that the men had to wade through slime on the ward floors. To make matters worse, the drinking supply for the hospital came from wells contaminated by the privies that were nearby. On top of all this, a hurricane struck the area, destroying many of the supplies. The harassed surgeons had to ask for help, even if the only help was from Nightingale. Nightingale and her nurses went to work cleaning the hospital, establishing a laundry, cooking the food, feeding the soldiers, and purveying the whole hospital, as well as caring for the sick and wounded. The soldiers responded to the nurses with gratitude, love, and affection, and the public, as it became aware of what she was doing, made Nightingale and her nurses heroines.

Nightingale was a determined, strong-willed woman, not easy to get along with, and she brooked no opposition from those under her command. One nurse brought charges against her that forced an investigation, but the nurse herself had to resign. Another party of nurses, led by Mary Stanley, refused to obey Nightingale and was eventually shunted off to another hospital. Despite these difficulties and her own high-handed methods, Nightingale's prestige continued to grow. The public worshipped her. She was a modern Joan of Arc who rapidly became one of the most written-about women in history.

Women had few heroines to match Florence Nightingale, and, inevitably, many a young girl wanted to become a nurse to do what Florence had done. Nursing was seen as a way for women to do something, to be somebody. Nursing was never the same. Troops at the Crimea had raised a special fund to honor her, the Nightingale Fund, and she used this to establish a nursing school at St. Thomas Hospital in London. With this, the Nightingale movement entered the civilian hospitals, and modern nursing had its origin. Note, however, that Nightingale, even in the stress of Crimea, was a lady. She did not confront the male physicians, she knew her place, and when the war was over, she slipped into England in order to avoid the crowds waiting to honor her. Although she was not particularly happy about the male dominance, she made it work. She reformed health care in the British army, founded a nursing school, established the public health nursing movement, and changed health care in India. She did all of this behind the scenes, mostly through male intermediaries who often received the credit. After her return from the Crimea, she deliberately sought obscurity, almost as if she believed the traditional statement that a woman's picture or story should only appear in the newspapers when she was engaged, when she was married, or when she died. After her return from the Crimea, she never made a public appearance, attended a public function, nor issued a public statement. Within a few years, most people assumed she was dead, but she was not. She was still working hard. She convinced Queen Victoria of the necessity for reform, but for either of these two women to be successful in any reform, they had to work through Parliament, and since women were not yet allowed to vote or sit in Parliament, this meant that they had to rely upon men. This need to work through indirection was part of being a nineteenth-century woman, and it had great influence on the ways in which nursing developed.

Because of the Nightingale image, nursing almost overnight was seen as an occupation for women. The American poet Longfellow had turned Florence into a mythical heroine in his poem that included the lines:

> A lady with a lamp shall stand
> In the great history of the land,
> A noble type of good,
> Heroic womanhood. (Longfellow, 1922)

NURSING IN THE AMERICAN CIVIL WAR

When the American Civil War broke out in 1861, women on both sides of the conflict inevitably volunteered their service. Put in charge of the northern nursing service was Dorothea Dix, a woman who had achieved fame for her work in improving prisons and in founding institutions for the mentally ill, but who had little knowledge of nursing. She was soon overwhelmed with applicants, although few had any training in nursing. To limit the applicants, she required that all enlistees be 30 years or older and be plain-looking women, whatever that might mean. One would-be nurse responded:

> I am in possession of one of your circulars, and will comply with all your requirements. I am plain looking enough to suit you, and old enough. I have no near relatives in the war, no lover there. I have never had a husband, and I am not looking for one. Will you take me? (Holland, 1895)

Several women emerged as heroines during the war; one of them, Mother Bickerdyke (1817–1901), is commemorated with a statue in her honor in Galesburg, Illinois.

Increasingly, there was a recognition of the need to extend nursing service into the growing hospital movement, and inevitably, nursing was thought of as something that only women could do. One of the things that happens to emerging groups, and women were an emerging group, is that they go into new or emerging occupations. Several new areas of potential employment emerged in the last part of the nineteenth century in what can be called the human services area: nursing, social work, library work, and elementary school teaching. Since all of these occupations demanded skills and abilities such as being supportive, helpful, and often dealt with children or with people who needed special help, they were regarded as natural for women. Women quickly moved to dominate them, at least for a time.

Nursing was especially appealing to many women in part because of the Florence Nightingale image, but also because many women saw it as a stepping stone to achieving greater equality for women. A good example of this latter viewpoint is Elizabeth Blackwell, the first woman to graduate from a medical college (in 1849). Blackwell spent much of her energies in the 1850s and 1860s trying to establish clinics for women, training nurses, and fighting to break through some of the barriers to women. Blackwell was strongly influenced by Nightingale and urged more women to study nursing rather than medicine, because the women physicians of her time were so "imperfectly trained" and would, in the long run, harm not only the medical profession but women's struggle for equality. Many women physicians, in fact, turned to nursing because of the barriers put in their way by the male medical establishment, as well as the fact that many came to regard it as more feminine than medicine.

The other emerging women professionals, such as social workers, librarians, or elementary school teachers, lacked the kind of independence that nurses had in their practice. This was because most graduate nurses did private practice or assumed managerial or teaching jobs for other nurses. Social work, although it had an authentic heroine in Jane Addams, always had to contend with the male establishment, and many of the more influential positions were held by men. It was men who were the heads of agencies or who served as probation officers or in other roles that came to be subsumed in the title of social worker. Librarians were generally women, but usually the key library administrators were men, and the professional librarians, mainly males in colleges and universities, had disproportionate influence over the profession. Elementary school teaching was as disproportionately female as nursing, but teachers' personal lives were more controlled than those of nurses, and in their professional organizations, they shared power with the male teachers in the secondary schools. Although nurses while in nursing school found their personal life rigidly supervised, once they entered private duty they had considerably more control over their own destiny than did women in almost any other occupation.

Nursing then offered an occupation in which a woman could remain "feminine," but still have some control over her own life, much more so than any other alternative occupation open to large numbers of women. It also had an heroic image given to it by Florence Nightingale, which was kept alive by other prominent nurses such as Dorothea Dix in the Civil War, and Lillian Wald at the beginning of the twentieth century. A nurse was someone who could do something important. No other occupation open to women could match its glamour, its image of dedication, its service, even its freedom.

REFERENCES

For more details:

Bullough, V.L. & Bullough, B. *The subordinate sex: A history of attitudes toward women.* Urbana, Ill.: University of Illinois Press, 1973; and New York: Penguin Books, 1974

Bullough, V.L. & Bullough, B. *The care of the sick: The emergence of modern nursing.* New York: Prodist, 1978.

Defoe, D. *A plan of the English commerce: Being a compleat prospect of the trade of this nation*, 2nd ed. 1730. New York: Augustus M. Kelley, 1967, pp. 90–92.

Defoe, D. *An essay: In which are given rules for expressing properly the principal passions and humours*, 1782. Quoted in *The genteel female: An anthology*. C.J. Furness (Ed.). New York: Knopf. 1931, p. 9.

Greg, M. in Pinchbeck, I. *Women workers and the industrial revolution 1750– 1850*. London: Frank Cass, 1969, pp. 315–316.

Holland, M.G. *Our army nurses*. Boston: Wilkins, 1895, p. 19.

Longfellow, H.W. *The complete poetical works of Longfellow*. Boston: Houghton-Mifflin, 1922, p. 197.

Woolstonecraft, M. *A vindication of the rights of women*. London: J.M. Dent, 1929, p. 23.

CHAPTER 2

Sex Discrimination and Nursing Education

Because modern nursing developed as a woman's profession, it suffered all the handicaps of women as well as problems of an emerging profession. One of the most obvious forms of discrimination practiced against women in the nineteenth century was denying them educational opportunities. Education, or at least advanced education, was a male privilege, and only a few women were able to break through this male bastion. Although there had been various female seminaries, the first coeducational institution of higher education in the United States was Oberlin College, founded in 1833, and higher education remained largely male until after the Civil War. The first woman's college, then known as Mount Holyoke Female Seminary, was established in 1837, but it technically was not chartered as a college until 1888. The other major women's colleges (now known as the seven sisters) were post-Civil War establishments: Vassar, 1865; Smith and Wellesley, 1875; Radcliffe, 1879; Bryn Mawr, 1885; Barnard, 1889. In short, nursing education at the time of its appearance was a real educational opportunity for large numbers of women. Yet none of the prestigious colleges for women ever established a nursing school (except Vassar during World War I), and, in fact, were not interested in training women for any kind of career. Instead, they concentrated on the liberal arts, and, in effect, denigrated the emerging women's professions. Teachers who also needed specialized education were, for the most part, taught in normal schools until after World War I. Normal schools were not colleges and, in most states, were the equivalent of high school. Only a few particularly enlightened colleges offered baccalaureate degrees to elementary school teachers. Social work was also out of the educational mainstream, and when it did enter the university, it did so as a graduate school in a few select universities. Although this made it socially more acceptable for upper-class women, it lacked the career opportunities for its graduates that nursing offered. Library work was also offered in special institutes during the last part of the nineteenth century and the first part of the twentieth century, and faced many of the handicaps that nursing did. In fact, many of the leading librarians never received a degree in library science but moved into the field from other areas.

Even if colleges had not been quite so discriminatory to women, however, nursing would have had difficulty in moving on to the college campus because medicine was not there. This leads us back to the interrelationship of nursing with medicine which is as important in shaping its direction as the fact that nursing was a woman's profession.

Although the United States had a number of medical colleges in the nineteenth century, most were colleges in name only. Few of the medical schools demanded as much as a high school diploma for admission, and none required a bachelor's degree. Many of the medical programs lasted only two years, and some lasted only six months. It was not until 1938 when the Johns Hopkins Medical School was founded, that medicine was established on a graduate level, and as late as 1905, only 5 of the 160 medical schools required any college work for admission. Although some of the colleges, such as Harvard Medical College, nominally had a college or university affiliation, the better medical schools were in fact part of the hospitals. Most medical colleges, however, lacked even that and were known as propriety schools, that is, private businesses run for profit, lacking university standards, facilities, or ideals. Americans who wanted the advanced training went to Europe for their medical education, a trend that continued until the end of the World War I, when American medical schools began to match and even surpass their European counterparts.

Medicine was also divided into various sects based on their theoretical approach to treatment: homeopathists, eclectics, osteopathists, allopathists. Many of the medical schools were little more than diploma mills without entrance requirements, hospital connections, or even teaching laboratories. Although some reforms had been introduced into medical education, public attention was effectively focused on the need for reform by the study of Abraham Flexner, who under the sponsorship of the Carnegie Foundation made recommendations to bring medicine to the status of a true graduate discipline. Flexner found that in 1910, only 680 (15.3%) of the 4,440 medical graduates had a bachelor's degree when they received their doctorate (Flexner, 1910), a number that rose to 43.5% by 1920. Most medical students received their bachelor's while studying for their doctorate. On a practical level, nursing training, as weak as it was in the nineteenth century, was often superior to the training of physicians because many medical students lacked actual hospital training until this century.

Perhaps to compensate for their lack of training, American physicians clung to the title of doctor. Doctor comes from the Latin word *docere*, meaning to teach, and it originally was given to those people who were qualified to teach in the universities. In Europe, there were severe restrictions on who could or could not be called a doctor, and to be termed a doctor implied a great honor. American physicians, in imitation, tended to call themselves doctors, although they lacked the training and education usually associated with such an advanced degree. Since most other college disciplines in the United States followed the English custom of issuing a master's degree as an advanced degree, this made physicians about the only doctors, and since every fly-by-night medical college claimed to issue a doctorate, the term came to be equated with physician. Even in Europe, most physicians at that time were holders of bachelor's degrees; the doctorate was reserved for the university professor. Seemingly, by claiming the doctorate, physicians were claiming educational backgrounds that they did not have, some indication of the insecurities of nineteenth-century American medicine.

Since physicians were trained in hospitals, it was inevitable that nurses be trained in hospitals as well. Although Marie Zakrzewska had founded a nursing school in 1860 and Elizabeth Blackwell had campaigned for more such schools to be affiliated with the women's medical colleges she attempted to found, it was not until 1873 that the English model training school established by Nightingale received a major impetus in the United States. Bellevue Hospital opened its school of nursing in May of 1873, followed in October by the Connecticut Training School in New Haven, and in November by the Boston Training School at Massachusetts General. All three schools, as well as most of those which followed in the next half-century, claimed to be based on the Nightingale model, but the use of the model was highly selective. Although some of the early training schools had funds to start, none of them were endowed, and many were not adequately financed. This meant that the hospitals expected work from the students, and the system followed much more of an apprenticeship model than an instructional one. Many hospitals did not even allow the minimal lectures series given at St. Thomas (weekly lectures), nor did the hospitals contract to employ their graduates after training as they did in England. Instead, they relied primarily on student nurses for running the hospitals, and nurses who graduated went on the registry to do private duty or went into nursing administration or education. At first, course work was only included in one of the years. The Illinois Training School for Nurses in 1877 was the first school to extend course work for the two years of nurse training. Early nursing classes often were rather heterogeneous, since the schools did not separate their students by prior education until after 1900, when the academically stronger schools stopped paying students a stipend. This led to some selective recruitment of more affluent and better prepared students into the stronger schools, since poorer students who often lacked the educational background needed the stipends.

From the first, there was a question of control of nursing education. In England, control clearly lay in the hands of the nurses. In this country, matters were not so clearly differentiated, and there always was much more hospital (read medical) control. In part, this was due to the influence of Johns Hopkins Hospital, which debated between the so-called Waltham Plan, (a physician-controlled nursing school in Waltham, Massachusetts, predating the Nightingale schools) and the Nightingale plan. Johns Hopkins set up a kind of compromise, with the nursing school placed under the hospital board of trustees rather than under a separate board of nursing education, but a nurse was made superintendent of the school and the hospital nursing service. This pattern was widely adopted, but actual nursing control was weak since physicians tended to become hospital board members and executives.

By the end of the nineteenth century, students in most American schools started with a two-month probationary period during which time they went to the wards to make beds and do other simple nursing tasks. At the end of this period, they were evaluated; if found satisfactory, they were allowed to wear the school uniform and attend lectures on applied science. Ward duty always took precedence over the lectures, however, as indicated by the following passage:

> Some knowledge of Anatomy, Physiology, Materia-Medica and Hygiene being found necessary, every training school has established a theoretical course which must, however, always be incidental to the ward work, though moving as it were hand in hand with it. Training schools for nurses can thus never be ranked as strictly educational . . . and the term "school" might be misleading, not indicating the fact that the time of the pupil nurses is largely spent in actual physical labor. (Hintz, 1898)

The usual hours on duty were from 7:00 A.M., to 7:00 P.M., with three hours off for dinner, study, and recreation. Night nurses, whose work was considered "less laborious," worked from 7:00 P.M. to 7:00 A.M., without time off.

Unfortunately for nursing education, the results of the new training schools appeared almost immediately in terms of patient benefits. Hospital administrators quickly found that establishing a nursing school not only improved hospital conditions but also reduced the cost of running the hospital, since so much of the work necessary to running of the hospital could be justified as part of nursing training. This included scrubbing the floors, cooking and serving the meals, as well as patient care. Medicine quickly delegated many of the more time-consuming tasks to nurses, and growth was rapid. In 1890 there were 15 nursing schools; in 1900 there were 432, an almost 3,000% increase.

Obviously, the system does not look the same to us today as it did to the would-be nurse in the 1890s. Where we might see exploitation, most early would-be nurses saw it as an opportunity for women to learn a useful occupation. In an 1898 survey of 325 nursing schools, there were only 8 general hospitals and 21 mental asylum schools that admitted male students. As the years passed, the proportion of males dropped even further. Moreover, nursing was about the only occupation that a poor girl could enter and get the necessary schooling. Colleges, even normal schools, were expensive. One biographer explained why Annie Goodrich, who later became Dean of the Yale School of Nursing, entered nursing in 1890 after her family had suffered financial setbacks:

> Annie, always an independent girl with a keen sense of responsibility, felt the need to be self-supporting. . . . She was quite honest with herself and admitted that she did not like nursing—far from it. She hated sickness and had a horror of death; nevertheless, since few vocational fields were open to women at the time she decided that entering the nursing profession was the best way to solve her problem. (Koch, 1951)

Many of the women who went into nursing were determined to upgrade themselves as well as their profession. This was harder to do than it seemed since they were caught in a "Catch 22." Colleges and universities did not give credit for nursing courses, yet the only way the women could gain educational credit and upgrade their standards was by attending college. This meant that those dedicated to nursing literally had to start their education over again since few had come to nursing with a college education, although many of them had a normal school diploma. Nurses met this problem both individually and collectively, and although the individual solutions helped in the short run, there was a strong feeling that all nursing had to upgrade itself.

In their search for solutions, a committee of the members of the Society of Superintendents of Nursing Schools, the forerunner of the National League for Nursing, made contact with Teachers College in New York, now a part of Columbia University. Although teachers' colleges themselves were stigmatized by the more traditional colleges, Teachers College had established itself as a national leader, and there was a willingness of its administration to help another educationally deprived group, nurses, raise their standards. An agreement was made effective for the fall of 1899 in which something called hospital economics, taught in the Department of Domestic Science, would be offered to nurses, if the Society raised the money for the instructor or guaranteed an enrollment of at least 12 students. In effect, this first effort was what today might be called either an extension program or continuing education. The members of the Society of Superintendents screened and admitted students, contributed $1,000 a year, and taught the course. Teachers College also allowed students to enroll in psychology, science, household economics, and biology. From such modest beginnings did modern collegiate nursing education in the United States and Canada start. Note that there were still no degrees in nursing.

Technically, the Teachers College experiment had been preceded by an attempt to establish a nursing program at Howard University in Washington, D.C. in 1893, but this effort, aimed at training black nurses, had failed. One of the difficulties nursing faced was that its organizational power was centered in the Northeast of the United States, while the logical place for it to gain an educational foothold was in the tax-supported state and municipal universities of the South, Midwest, and West. There were, however, problems in these institutions since many of the state institutions were located in small towns, away from major hospitals. In fact, the medical schools, which increasingly became attached to such universities, were often in different cities than the main campus of the university. The University of Illinois Medical School, for example, was in Chicago, while the University itself was in Champaign-Urbana. There were, however, some state universities in major cities, and it was in one of these, the University of Minnesota in Minneapolis, in 1909, that the first basic nursing program with a university affiliation was started. The program, however, was strongly hospital-oriented, and although students were required to meet university admission standards, they worked a 56-hour week on the hospital wards during their student period. Instead of receiving a degree, they received a diploma after three years, but they did receive college credit for some of their work.

In 1916, the University of Cincinnati took the next logical step and established a degree option by giving both the diploma and a baccalaureate degree. The degree, however, took five years. In 1917, Columbia University put together a five-year program in conjunction with Presbyterian Hospital in New York, and a similar program started in San Francisco, at the University of California. These five-year degree programs included two years of basic sciences at the university, two years of nursing experience at the hospital, and one year of special training in public health or education. By 1923, there were 17 schools with degree options, all except Columbia-Presbyterian, in the western or southern parts of the United States.

Students who wanted to go for advanced training went on in education for the most part, since graduate schools of education were more likely to accept the credits of nurses who graduated from the nursing colleges. Graduate programs for nursing developed at the University of Chicago, Case Western Reserve, Catholic University, and Teachers College. Most were closely allied to educational programs, and there was an emphasis on educational techniques, curriculum modification, which further separated the nurses with advanced degrees from those who did not have them. This was because they more or less left nursing for administration or teaching, and their advanced courses had little nursing content. Graduate degrees in nursing itself did not appear until after World War II, except for the special ones issued by Yale University and, for a time, by Case Western Reserve, but neither of these degrees required a bachelor's in nursing as an entrance requirement. The result was that few nurses learned basic research techniques, partly because education as a whole was not concerned with research and treated it as something reserved for the Ph.D. not the Ed.D. Nurses who did not want to go on to graduate work in an academic subject such as physiology or sociology had to make up for what their undergraduate training lacked in these areas, because few programs gave credit for their courses with nursing content. Again as in so many other areas, nursing had to pull itself up by its own bootstraps, so to speak, although in this area, it began to receive help from the federal government in the aftermath of World War II.

REFERENCES

For more details:

Bullough, V.L. & Bullough, B. *Care of the sick: The emergence of modern nursing.* New York: Prodist, 1978.

Flexner, A. *Medical education in the United States and Canada.* New York: Carnegie Foundation for Advancement of Teaching, 1910, p. 291.

Flexner, A. Medical education in the United States. *Journal of the American Medical Association,* 1922, **79**, 692–696.

Hintz, A.A. The training term. In J. Hodson (Ed.), *How to become a trained nurse.* New York: William Abbatt, 1898, p. 19.

Koch, H.B. *Militant angel.* New York: Macmillan, 1951, p. 14.

CHAPTER 3

Economics of the Profession

Although the sex segregation so common in nursing gave women the opportunity for leadership within the profession, it had the disadvantage of blocking upward mobility beyond the segregated system. Although nurses could become directors of nursing or deans of nursing schools, probably the highest ranking positions within the profession, they could not become directors of hospitals or presidents of universities. In this sense, nurses were like blacks who suffered under a different kind of segregation, in which advancement was primarily limited to those institutions serving the black community.

The disadvantage of the segregated system, in fact, becomes obvious when nurses are compared to blacks; success was possible as long as they accepted the limits put on them by the system. Since nurses were part of a hierarchial health care system, they had to be careful not to overstep their bounds. But because nurses were women, they also had to preserve their feminine image of the helpful girl Friday, or risk being ostracized by others within the hierarchy. Other more male-dominated occupations within the system could be more demanding, more aggressive, more obnoxious, if you will, and gain concessions, but nurses who made demands were accused of being witches or bitches or some other less flattering terms. The result was often a failure by the high-status members of the health establishment to recognize what nurses do, and as a result, nursing itself was downgraded and underpaid compared with other health occupations.

Part of the difficulty is that females traditionally have been socialized to act in certain ways to men; to play what could be described as a male-female game. The rules for this traditional game have been described most effectively by the anti-feminist Helen

Andelin, in her book *Fascinating Womanhood* (n.d.). Mrs. Andelin, the name she prefers to use, urged women not to confront a man directly, never denigrate his masculinity, and never contradict him. Instead, she advocated the use of feminine wiles, even to acting the role of a little girl who stamps her feet or shakes her curls, and, if necessary, breaks into tears when she is frustrated (Andelin, n.d.). Although nurses never quite adopted the ideal woman of Mrs. Andelin's book as their role prescription, they did play their own version of the female-male game.

A poem that ran in a nineteenth-century nursing journal included the lines:

> Nurses moving quietly,
> Voices hushed in awe,
> All things silent waiting,
> Obedient to the law
> That we have heard so often,
> But I'll repeat once more
> All things must be in order
> When Doctor's on the floor.
> (*Trained Nurse and Hospital Review, 1896*)

Nurses were taught that physician's word was law, that they were to stand when the physician entered the ward or the room, and that it would be rude for a nurse to speak to a physician openly and honestly or to even offer suggestions about the nursing care of the patients, a subject about which they knew much more than he did. In fact, if a patient asked a question, the answer to which the nurse was well aware, she had always to respond with, "Ask the doctor."

Such behavior is contrary to the reality of the nursing situation. Ordinarily, the physician only sees the hospitalized patient for a few minutes each day; he has to depend on someone for the information and this someone is usually the nurse. Nurses observe the patient's condition hour after hour; they have a chance to hear what he or she has to say. They know when to intervene and when not to intervene and when to ask the physician for permission to intervene. Under the rules of the old doctor-nurse game, however, nurses had to pretend that they never diagnosed or made recommendations. The game was well described by the psychiatrist Leonard Stein in 1967. He was fascinated by the strange way in which nurses made suggestions to physicians so that both the physician and the nurse could pretend recommendations had not been made. He called the pattern a transactional neurosis (Stein, 1967).

A good example of this behavior was observed by one of the

authors of this book in her supervision of students on a medical floor. Many of the patients on the ward, seriously ill cardiac patients, received digitalis or related synthetic drugs. The dosage for these drugs, as all nurses know, has to be adjusted to the individual patient, and since the therapeutic dose is close to the toxic dose, the patient must be observed carefully for symptoms of toxicity, particularly when first being digitalized. The conscientious and knowledgeable nurses on the ward observed the patients for symptoms of toxicity as indicated by a slow pulse rate, nausea, or depression. Nurses could read the monitors and readily identify the characteristic cardiac arrhythmias that suggested this type of toxicity. When they noted symptoms of a developing toxicity, they would immediately withhold the drug and then notify the physician, not of their actions, but of their observations. In fact, they would not tell the physician that they had noted symptoms suggesting toxicity. They would simply report the discrete symptoms as if they did not understand the implications. The doctor would then tell them to withhold or lessen the digitalis dosage, and they would thank him for the "order."

If, however, the doctor was a new resident, or for other reasons did not appear to understand the implications of what the nurse was reporting, they would "accidentally" later drop the information about the symptoms in a conversation with a third-year resident or an attending physician, and the hapless young physician would be in trouble for not acting on the nurses' observation. Thus, even though the nurses had made a decision and acted, they avoided, at all costs, the responsibility for their decisions.

Although we criticize nurses for doing this, those nurses who attempted to break out of the system were often punished. This system and its consequences even shows up in fictionalized accounts. One of the more famous series of medical novels is the Dr. Kildare series, which has also served as the basis of a number of movies and television plays and series. One of the key characters is the termagant Dr. Gillespie, originally played by Lionel Barrymore in the movie productions, who consistently puts down nurses (Brand, 1940). In one such account, the nurse asks the physician what certain tests revealed about a patient going for surgery. His response:

> He brushed her off impatiently, almost rudely. "I'm not in the habit of confiding in our nursing staff about things which can't possibly concern them. Shall we leave it at that?"
> "Certainly, doctor." (Frazer, 1964)

In yet another story, a nurse is transferred to care for a patient at the doctor's request. She comes in on her evening off to begin the case. Soon afterward, the doctor appears and begins to shout:

> "You were to phone me a half hour ago, nurse. I received no call. . . ."
>
> Veronica's lips tightened. "No-one told me I was supposed to phone you, doctor."
>
> He said, his voice edgy with sarcasm, "Can you read nurse? It's written on the chart."
>
> . . . She flushed. "I'm sorry, doctor, I guess I missed seeing it."
>
> Veronica felt anger rising in her. He had no right . . . ! She hadn't been careless! Still . . . she should have seen that notation. She succeeded in holding back her anger. "No, doctor." "Next time," he said, "see if you can perform your functions as a nurse, the way they should be performed!"
>
> Veronica's lips tightened, but she managed to say past their trembling, "Yes, doctor." (Brenna, 1962)

Such patterns of subservience and feminine submissiveness led to an undervaluing of the contributions of nurses. This is reflected in the salaries paid nurses. This salary problem was clearly demonstrated in the court case brought by the nurses employed by the City and County of Denver, known as *Lemons v. Denver,* and carried by the Denver attorney Craig S. Barnes. Taking jobs held primarily by males and comparing them to nurses, it was demonstrated in every case that male occupations included in the city roster, regardless of the educational training required, paid more than occupations that were predominantly female (Barnes, 1980). The 100% male classification jobs, for example, averaged $1,593 per month, while the 100% female classes averaged only $1,091. Some examples of these groups are indicated in Table 1. Starting salaries for male-dominated jobs were found to be consistently higher, even though the male-dominated jobs required comparable or lower qualifications in the areas of education, experience, and supervisory responsibility. In one comparison of 35 exclusively male jobs, all of which required fewer years of education and experience and the same or less supervisory responsibility as a floor nurse, the male classes were paid more than both the floor nurse and the head nurse.

For the trial, a professional evaluation of traditional job worth was done. This technique computed factors such as physical effort, job complexity, responsibility, accountability, supervision exercised, and working conditions. At the same level of job worth, it was determined that as the number of males in a specific classification increased, the salary also increased. Further, the sex of the incumbent uniformly was

TABLE 1. SEX SEGREGATION: INEQUALITIES IN INCOME IN THE CITY
AND COUNTY OF DENVER

Job Classification	Monthly Starting Salary ($)		Salary Difference ($)	
	1978	1979	Month	Year
Graduate nurse I (beginning)	929.00	1,064.00		
100% Male Jobs Classifications				
Sign painter	1,245.00	1,361.00	297.00	3,564.00
Painter	1,088.00	1,191.00	127.00	1,524.00
Tree trimmer	1,040.00	1,164.00	100.00	1,200.00
Tire serviceman	1,017.00	1,113.00	49.00	588.00
Parking meter repairman	994.00	1,113.00	49.00	588.00

determined to be the significant factor in salary differences (Bullough & Bullough, 1982; Barnes, 1980).

Judge Fred Winner of the 10th Circuit Federal District Court, in ruling against the nurses, acknowledged that the evidence effectively indicated that nursing, as an occupation, had been discriminated against, but he stated that if he had ruled in favor of nurses, there was the potential of "disrupting the entire economic system of the United States of America" (Bullough, 1978). In 1980, the Supreme Court chose not to rehear the case, but they did rule in a case reaching the court about the same time, and dealing with women prison guards. In this second case, the court ruled that inequality between the sexes had been demonstrated, and ordered the state to make redress. By 1983 the Denver nurses had been vindicated. The doctrine of comparable worth was accepted in a Tacoma, Washington case by a Federal judge, and if this is upheld by the Supreme Court, nursing will change radically (*New York Times,* Nov. 1, 1983).

The simple fact of being a woman has traditionally had a significant effect on wages and salaries. Complicating the inequalities of nursing salaries is the historical fact that nursing has not participated vigorously in collective bargaining. In 1947, the National Labor Relations Act (Taft-Hartley) specifically excluded nonprofit health care institutions from its provisions. The result was that hospitals were under no obligation to negotiate with their workers. As a result, only 15% of the health care workers were organized by the end of 1974 when the National Labor Relations Act was revised. Nurses therefore had to overcome not only the fact that they were women but that they were discriminated against by official policy. Still, it has to be said that the existence of such barriers was partly due to a lack of militancy shown by nurses, a problem also tied to their feminine identity.

Perhaps the best illustration of this attitude is the Model Practice Act adopted in 1955 by the Board of Directors of the American Nurses' Association (ANA), which seriously handicapped the expansion of nursing when it was accepted by legislators in 21 states. Professional nursing practice was defined as follows:

> The term, "practice of professional" nursing means the performance for compensation, of any acts in the observation, care and counsel of the ill, injured or infirm or in the maintenance of health or prevention of illness of others, or in the supervision and teaching of other personnel or the administration of medications and treatments as prescribed by a licensed physician or a licensed dentist; requiring substantial specialized judgment and skill and based on knowledge and application of principles of biological, physical and social science. The foregoing shall *not be deemed to include any acts of diagnosis or prescription of therapeutic or corrective measures.* (Bullough, 1980; ANA, 1955)

The fascinating thing about the underlined disclaimer is that it was not made by the American Medical Association but by the American Nurses' Association. Although it might be a reasonable assumption that the nurses felt the disclaimer necessary to avoid medical opposition to the new practice acts of that period, there is little evidence of overt pressure by medical people. Being good women, the nurses surrendered before any battle over boundaries could occur.

Even before the disclaimer was adopted, some nurses, particularly those in university positions, were evolving an ideological position, trying to separate the function of nurses from the function of physicians. What these nurses did was emphasize the social and psychological components of nursing often at the expense of the physical and then claim jurisdiction over the social and psychological. Ultimately, however, the major reason for the disclaimer, at least in our opinion, was alienation or what might be called anticipatory self-discriminatory behavior of nurses. Rather than risk a rebuff or a possible boundary dispute with medicine, nurses almost unconsciously decided to avoid admitting their role in the patient care decision-making process. Similar patterns of anticipatory self-discrimination are a fairly common phenomenon among minority groups; the ghetto walls are often as well policed from the inside as from the outside, and in the past, feelings of powerlessness and fear have often prevented people from challenging discriminatory practices.

Moreover nurses had few male allies. Men who were interested in becoming nurses not only had to face the low salaries, but also had to overcome the stereotypical feminine image and the very real feminine action-pattern in dealing with the world. In addition, many had to confront publicly the issue of sex preference long before being "gay" was widely accepted. Since nursing was so strongly identified in ideal and in action with women, men who went into it were usually categorized as homosexual, whether or not they were gay. Thus, it took a strong-willed individual willing to accept his own sexuality to deal with the biases and prejudices so endemic to being a male nurse. Those men who did, however, often emerged into leadership positions fairly rapidly because they had not been so acclimatized to playing the subordinate role.

Nursing, however, is changing, and probably the most important and significant movement affecting change in nursing has been the woman's movement of the 1970s. Whatever else the movement might have accomplished, and however initially it denigrated nurses, it gave permission to women to challenge some of the age-long discrimination. Nurses were in the forefront of those doing this. The movement also made it easier for men to enter into nursing if only because the male and female role models became less rigid than they had been in the past. Approximately 6% of the students now in nursing schools are men (National League for Nursing 1981). Coinciding with the new militancy of women, in general, were changes in the labor legislation which allowed nurses to organize, and a realization that they had to expand their turf to meet the threat of the newly emerging physician's assistant movement aimed entirely at men. Either nurses were going to be permanent girl Fridays, or they had to meet the challenge. Reluctantly, and with considerable ambivalence, they met the challenge, aided by the rapid expansion of the health care industry. New specialties emerged or were re-established, often with the support of the medical profession who, in their increasingly narrow specialization, were willing to delegate more and more to nurses. Among the specialties that emerged in the 1970s were nurse practitioners, midwives, anesthetists, and clinical specialists. In the process, nurses found themselves forced to make decisions and take responsibility or lose out. The willingness to change was marked in most states by a new round of nurse practice acts that gave nurses new accountability and a willingness to accept their right to intervene for the patient's welfare (Bullough, 1980). All these changes, however, raised new issues.

REFERENCES

ANA board approves a definition of nursing practice. *American Journal of Nursing,* December 1955, **55,** 1474.

Andelin, H. *Fascinating womanhood.* Santa Barbara, Calif.: Pacific Press, n.d.

Barnes, C. Denver: A case study. In B. Bullough (Ed.), *The law and the expanding nursing role.* New York: Appleton-Century-Crofts, 1980, pp. 125–137.

Brand, M. *Dr. Kildare's crisis.* New York: Dell, 1940.

Brenna, A. *Nurse's dormitory.* New York: Prestige Books, 1962.

Bullough, B. *The law and the expanding nursing role.* New York: Appleton-Century-Crofts, 1980.

Bullough, B. & Bullough, V. Nursing as a profession. In P.L. Stewart & M.G. Cantor (Eds.), *Varieties of work.* Beverly Hills, Calif.: Sage Publications, 1982, pp. 213–224.

Frazer, D. *Nurse with a past.* New York: Pocket Books, 1964.

Hershey, R.D. Woman's pay fight shifts to comparable worth. *New York Times,* November 1, 1983, A15.

National League for Nursing. *Nursing data book* 1980. New York: NLN, 1981.

Stein, L. The doctor-nurse game. *Archives of General Psychiatry,* 1967, **16,** 699–703.

Trained Nurse and Hospital Review. 1896, **16,** 90.

CHAPTER 4

Organizational Problems in a Woman's Profession

Because so many nurses were women, much of the battle that nurses have had to fight to gain recognition has been for women's rights. Perhaps this accounts for the fact that many of the most influential women in American life have been nurses. On a recent list of 20 of the most influential women in the history of the United States, three of the women were nurses: Lillian Wald, Margaret Sanger, and Emma Goldman. If the list had been confined to women who had made their reputation for their own activities rather than being given added significance because they were an important person's wife, such as Abigail Adams, the wife of our second president, the nursing representation might well have been even more significant. American history, in fact, is full of significant nurses or women who acted as nurses, such as Dorothy Dix, Clara Barton, Louisa May Alcott, Sister Elizabeth Kenny, St. Elizabeth Seton. Most of the heroines of the past 150 years have been nurses, and their ranks include women as diverse as Mother Bickerdyke, the Civil War heroine, to Clara Maas, who gave her life in the fight to eliminate yellow fever in the aftermath of the Spanish-American War. It was a French nurse, Genevieve de Galard, who made headlines in the 1960s at Dienbienphu in Vietnam. Mary Breckinridge opened up the hill country of Kentucky to public health. The list could go on for several chapters. Nurses, in fact, have probably gone more places and done more things than any other single group of women.

As an organized group of women, nurses have also been signifi-cant. Nurses organized the first major professional association for women, edited and published the first professional magazine by women, and were the first major professional group to integrate black and white members. It is still the best integrated at every level of any national organization. Deans of nursing remain the most visible token women in college and university administration, and nurses are the ranking women officers in most of the armed forces.

In spite of the long list of successful battles that nurses have fought and won for women, and the list would fill several additional pages, most of the bibliographies dealing with women's history ignore nurses. As indicated earlier, no high-status women's college ever had more than a short-lived nursing school, and when the feminist movement took note of nursing in the early 1970s, it was, for the most part, to put them down. In fact, one of the early slogans of the women's movement was for women to encourage their daughters to avoid nursing and become a physician instead.

This ignorance of nursing by the women's movement of the past few decades was not just a put-down by the feminists. It was partly a response to a coping mechanism that nurses, and probably a number of other women-dominated groups, followed throughout much of the twentieth century. In retrospect, what seemed to have happened is that women, denied a place in the male world, made their own place in the female world. Since the feminist movement, at least in its early phases, was an attempt to get women more into the male world, the world where they believed "real" power existed, and   turn their backs on the ghettoized female world, nurses and all similar women's groups were simply shunted aside. Some nurses contributed to this (Muff, 1982).

Although nurses who had received national and international recognition are listed above, the traditional heroines of organized nursing have not been Sanger, Wald, or Goldman who fought for and gained power in the world at large, but the women who did their fighting within nursing to help it advance: Adelaide Nutting, Lavina Dock, Isabel Hampton Robb, Annie Goodrich, and others. These women, however, are generally unknown to the nonnursing world and were ignored by the feminist-oriented historians.

Many years ago the sociologist Robert Merton described the difference in professional power between those who sought power at a local or parochial setting, and those who sought power at a national or cosmopolitan level. In terms of professional advancement, it was the cosmopolitan recognition that counted most, although there was considerable satisfaction in being recognized as important at the local level by those who sought such recognition. Thus, the local college professor who achieved a reputation as a good teacher or a good local administrator was probably loved by his students and faculty, but the power and prestige went to the professor who read papers at national meetings, engaged in committee work at the national level, and whose work was well-known both within and without the profession, and was able to influence significant segments of the population (Merton, 1966). Merton's dichotomy is useful in dealing with the male professions, but it is not so useful in dealing with nursing or with other women's groups. This is because nurses as women were denied power at the cosmopolitan level of being able to influence the world at large; instead, large numbers concentrated on influencing nursing. In a sense, this was an attempt to gain internal influence in areas where external influence was difficult, if not impossible, to achieve. Thus, their achievements and abilities were recognized by those who belonged to nursing organizations but not to the world outside of the profession. In this sense, Wald, Sanger, Goldman, Kenny, et al., were externally oriented nurses who chose to work in the world at large, while those recognized as leaders of the profession were those who worked from within. The feminists who put down nursing were externalists and knew little and cared little about the internal world of nursing.

It was not just ignorance of the internal leaders, however, that contributed to the put-down of nurses by the feminist movement, but also the very real difficulty of the internalist success for the feminist movement as a whole. This is because success in the internal world of women might well demand different qualities than in the external world so controlled by men in the past. This, in retrospect, has complicated the ability of nurses in communicating the very real issues about which they are concerned to the public at large.

As a college administrator who is also a nurse, the male co-author of this book often finds himself drawn into conversation with college administrators about those "crazy nurses" on their faculty. Many college administrators seem to lack understanding of what nurses want or why there seems to be so much difficulty with their nursing departments or schools. Undoubtedly, part of the difficulty is a simple male unwillingness to deal with some of the predominantly female groups on their faculty, but it is also due, in part, to the fact that nursing goals are still deeply influenced by professional associations that have not yet come to terms with the nonnursing world.

Nursing has been a women's profession, and there was in the past a basic dichotomy between the regular nurse and the nursing leaders. Although this is partly an age differential between the older and younger nurses, such an age disparity is common to almost all organized professions. This disparity in nursing was accentuated because comparatively few of the women who became nurses took any kind of leadership role in the professional development. This was simply because nurses were women, and in the recent past, the nursing work force was dominated by young unmarried women, while the organizational power structure was dominated by older unmarried women. Since most nurses were forced to leave nursing when they married, this meant that the organizational structure was in the hands of those who, for one reason or another, made nursing organizational work the focus of their lives. This was not necessarily a deliberate attempt of the unmarried to exclude the married, but a fact of life for most women. Quite simply, married women were not allowed to teach, serve as public librarians, nurses, social workers, or secretaries until well into the twentieth century. Those employed in governmental agencies at both the state and local levels were usually forced by law to leave. The few married women who did retain jobs in these professions made their occupational role secondary to their domestic roles of wife and mother. Inevitably, if a profession was to grow and develop, in fact simply survive, it took the dedicated devotion of women who could both work and give their time to the profession, mainly the older single women. This fact further escalated the isolation between the "regular" world and the nursing world since single women themselves were stigmatized by society. All kinds of roadblocks were put in their path by society to prevent them from asserting themselves effectively in the external cosmopolitan world.

Even if the legal and social strictures against married working women had been relaxed, working conditions in nursing favored the unmarried women. Those hospitals and institutions that employed women had a 12-hour day until the beginning of World War II. Moreover, nurses were often required to live in a nurse's home, guaranteeing ready access to the hospital for emergencies. The more specialized jobs such as nursing education, public health nursing, or school nursing usually were legally restricted to the unmarried woman. The one job in which a married woman could work was a private duty nurse's job, through the registry, taking care of families or individuals in time of illness. A nurse on the registry waited her turn for a case, and if for family or other reasons she was unable to accept the one that came up for her assignment, she had to start the wait over again. Thus, even the registry worked against the married woman.

Inevitably there was a distinction within nursing between those who were planning to make a career of nursing, and those who were in it for a short term. Ultimately this distinction was between the lesbian woman or the dedicated spinster, and the woman who visualized herself as a wife and mother. Any survey of the biographies of the dominant leaders of nursing demonstrates that until after World War II, there were almost no married women influential in the internal affairs of nursing, although there were some who had been married and widowed or divorced. In the early years of nursing, the only influential leader to be married was Isabel Hampton Robb, and she was strongly denounced by her colleagues for her fall from the single state. Adelaide Nutting, one of her contemporaries, even went so far as to state that Robb had betrayed nursing by getting married. Although Robb remained active in nursing affairs, she no longer nursed. Her wealth and social position was such that she could dedicate her spare time to the organizational activities of nursing. In spite of this dedicated service, her nursing colleagues never quite forgave her for her marriage.

Nursing leaders were not only overwhelmingly single, but significant numbers had entered nursing as older women, i.e., in their late 20s or early 30s, and had already decided not to marry. Nursing was visualized by most of them as an opportunity for independence and advancement, and their commitment to nursing had come only after rejection of most of the other alternatives. Many of these latecomers to nursing also saw nursing as a way in which they could work for the advancement of women, since the struggles of nursing were part of the fight for women to gain influence in the male-dominated hospitals and colleges and the world at large. The more power these single women gained in the profession and in the educational institutions (most of which were hospital schools until World War II), the less contact they had with actual nursing, which remained an occupation for young unmarried women. Their power, in a sense, was built on other women, and although they negotiated with the male-dominated world, nursing policies often developed independently of this world, and the outsider often had difficulty in understanding it. Since decisions were often arrived at more or less autocratically, if only because power was limited to the small group of dedicated professionals, the decisions often reflected the special needs and interests of this group rather than those regarded as more pressing by the hospital nurse or even the registry nurse (Bullough, in press).

Further contributing to a narrow internalist view of nursing was the fact that the organizational leadership during the first half of the twentieth century was concentrated in a few urban areas in the Northeast: New York, Boston, Baltimore, with Chicago as a midwest center. Educationally, there were strong ties of the leadership to Teachers College (TC) in New York, and when nurses did go on to higher degrees, they usually went to TC. The result was a general agreement in goals by the internalist-oriented leadership who increasingly were also cut off by what was happening in the rest of the country. The connection with TC meant that most of the advanced nursing education dealt with how to teach nursing rather than encouraging scientific or scholarly investigation of the kind carried out in the various disciplines. Although TC was an outstanding school of education, probably the best in the country, education itself was stigmatized by the other disciplines, and nursing, while upgrading itself by its affiliation with TC, also was being stigmatized by it. Not infrequently, the result was a kind of ghetto mentality in which nurses tended to find the solution in curriculum revision. Since a major part of the course work for advanced degrees in education deal with curriculum planning and innovation, it was perhaps inevitable that nursing periodically went through mass curriculum changes. In fact, nursing seemingly has had more major curriculum changes than any other academic discipline on college campuses.

Challenges and changes to this tradition came primarily from the West and Midwest, where collegiate nursing schools appeared in the state universities and colleges, a kind of institution which was either nonexistent or not important in most of the Northeast until after World War II. The first effect of the western challenge was to strengthen the internalist view of nursing since the eastern leadership, where the nursing organizations were headquartered, developed an "old girl" network that had a "common" professional ambition and sense of direction, and that managed to dominate nursing through control of the key professional committees, such as those devoted to accrediting, which remained independent of the membership.

In the rapid expansion of nursing following the World War II period and with the changing social conditions for women, the composition of the profession changed both socially and economically. Nursing education was upgraded and salaries improved. Barriers against married women gradually disappeared, and women found it possible to combine a career and marriage and family without being socially ostracized by the world at large. The generation that came of age in the postwar period when such movement for women was possible, however, are now in their 40s and early 50s. In general, they tend to be much more externalist than their earlier generations, and the result is a lessening of distinctions between professions dominated by women and other professions. This change, however, has not been soon enough to overcome some of the handicaps of the previous internalist view. The most notable example is the growth of trade unions for nursing. In part, these unions got a stronghold because organized nursing, at first, was reluctant to enter into collective bargaining. Even with those state associations, more "willing-to-do-so" nurses often were handicapped because of the comparative lack of women with bargaining experience. The next few years will be crucial in determining the organizational directions that nursing will take. The issues are discussed in section 3.

REFERENCES

Bullough, V. Nurses and politics. *Women and politics.* 1984, in press.

Merton, R. Patterns of influence. In P. Lazarsfeld and F. Stanton (Eds.), *Communications research 1948–49.* New York: Harper, 1948; reprinted in Merton, R. *Social theory and social structure,* rev. New York: Free Press, 1966, pp. 441–474.

Muff, J. Why doesn't a smart girl like you go to medical school? In J. Muff, *Socialization, sexism, and stereotyping.* St. Louis: Mosby, 1982, pp. 178–189.

Section II

CURRENT TRENDS AND ISSUES IN HISTORICAL PERSPECTIVE

CHAPTER 5

Nursing Education

The history of modern nursing is usually dated from the establishment of the St. Thomas Hospital Training School by Florence Nightingale. This simple fact serves to emphasize how important nursing education has been to nursing and to nurses. Seemingly, each development in nursing has been demarcated by some basic changes in nursing education, and the struggle for educational opportunity has been the dominant theme in the history of American nursing.

Nurses, as indicated in an earlier chapter, have traditionally labored under a handicap in raising their education level, both because they were women and because the health professions themselves are hierarchical, and physicians at the top of the pyramid have usually had very mixed feelings about well-educated nurses. Other factors also were important.

COLLEGIATE EDUCATION FOR NURSES

Even though there were opportunities for women to attend college in the United States when the Nightingale Training Schools were established here in 1873, very few colleges admitted women, and it was very unlikely they would establish anything such as a nursing school. Teacher training, at least of elementary teachers, was confined to the normal schools, and the only subject matter specifically designed for women was home economics, which was struggling to get a foothold in a few colleges. The women's colleges, which on the surface ought to have been more receptive, steered clear of vocational and professional training and instead concentrated on the liberal arts.

While women's colleges offered intellectual challenges to their students, they also visualized most of their students as potential wives and mothers and not as long-time working women. There was also a class difference between the women's colleges and the nurse training schools in that the colleges tended to be upper middle class, and those women aiming for a career tended to look to the long-established professions while nursing schools attracted primarily lower middle-class students.

The fact that most of the early nursing schools were located on the east coast areas of the United States also made it difficult to gain a foothold in the colleges. Most of the sexually integrated state-supported colleges and universities were in the West, Midwest, and South. This made it less likely that nursing would be able to move programs into colleges and universities or even to affiliate with colleges and universities. Similarly, state-supported medical schools with university affiliations appeared most often in the same sections of the United States, and while medical schools moved from private hospitals to private universities in the East, these same private universities often had barriers to women and were too status conscious to accept nursing students.

Another factor handicapping nursing from moving into colleges and universities was the economic benefits accruing to a hospital that established a Nightingale Training School. Still, women wanted the kind of educational opportunities that nursing offered, and they flocked to the nursing schools. The rapid growth of nursing schools allowed medicine to become more specialized, if only because the physician could delegate more and more tasks to nurses. Inevitably this led to a raising of educational standards for physicians and an increase in their income and status. It would, in fact, be fair to state that it was only because nursing education moved into the hospitals that medical education could move into the university (Bullough & Bullough, 1978).

Cut off from a college education through the front door, nursing found entrance at the back door. The beginning of higher education for nurses dates from what today we could call an extension course taught by the newly organized Superintendents Society (forerunner of the modern National League for Nursing) through the aegis of Teachers College, Columbia University. Dean James Russell agreed to allow the nurses to offer a course, providing they would guarantee an enrollment of 12 persons or pay $1,000 a year. In the end, members of the society screened and admitted students, contributed $1,000, and taught the course. In 1905, Adelaide Nutting was hired by Teachers College to direct the program. Not until 1910 when the program was endowed by Helen Hartley Jenkins did it become firmly entrenched (Christy, 1969; Cunningham, 1959). The program, however, was in education, not in nursing itself.

The first basic nursing program in a collegiate institution was started in 1909 at the University of Minnesota. It was, however, not a degree program. Although students enrolled in the program were required to meet university standards for admission and classwork, they also had to work 56 hours a week on the hospital ward. After three years they received a diploma from the University, not a degree (Gray, 1960). This modest alliance with academia was copied by a few other tax-supported universities, including Cincinnati, Indiana, Virginia, and Washington (MacDonald, 1965). Finally in 1916, Cincinnati took the next logical step and established a degree option.

EFFORTS TO IMPROVE THE HOSPITAL TRAINING PROGRAMS

Whereas these pioneer collegiate programs are important, they were not the only significant developments of this period in the eventual reform of nursing education. Important also were the efforts of nurses to raise the overall standards of education in diploma programs (Munson & Stevens, 1934). In 1917 the National League of Nursing Education (NLNE) issued its *Standard Curriculum for Schools of Nursing.* This report outlined a three-year sequence including course work in basic sciences and nursing, clinical experience caring for patients with medical, surgical, obstetrical, pediatric, and if possible, special disease conditions. The committee recommended that pupil nurses work no more than eight hours a day and advocated that high school graduation be required for admission (NLNE, 1917). The curriculum was revised and updated in 1927 (NLNE, 1927) and 1937 (NLNE, 1937). Since the standards outlined in these guides were not adhered to in most training schools, they might better be regarded as calls for change. They were also considered somewhat controversial. There were many nurses who felt that it was more important to preserve the old emphasis on devotion to duty, which they felt was the cornerstone of the Nightingale model. They argued that the abandonment of the 12-hour day for students and hospital nurses or the 20-hour day for private duty nurses was an abandonment of the ideals of the profession. This meant that educational reformers struggled not only against the powerful hospital establishment and the conservative physicians but also against some members of their own profession (Jamme, 1919; Stewart, 1919).

THE GOLDMARK REPORT

Consequently, nurses who wanted to improve educational standards sought outside validation of their ideas through a series of major reports written by researchers, who were not nurses, backed up by committees made up of distinguished persons. These reports are fascinating, not only as coping mechanisms but also as historical documents. They tend to reflect the thinking of the nursing leadership group at the time they were published, although these ideas were often attributed to the professional researcher who was hired to spearhead the report. Medicine had first used the report strategy as a reform platform with the Flexner report of 1910 (Flexner, 1910). Nursing's first major use of the approach was in 1923, when the Goldmark report was issued. The committee that sponsored it had been established in 1918 with funds from the Rockefeller Foundation. The committee's first charge was to investigate the educational opportunities open to nurses who wanted to work in the community, but its members decided that the hospital training programs should be improved in order to provide a better basis for postgraduate public health courses.

Josephine Goldmark was hired as secretary and researcher for the committee. She did an empirical study of 49 community agencies and 23 of the better nursing schools. While the data from this survey were important, they were used primarily as a springboard and documentation for committee conclusions. Other literature and the strongly held opinions of the group members were also considered.

A series of recommendations for strengthening hospital nursing schools were issued. The committee agreed with Adelaide Nutting, who had long argued that the basic problem was a lack of adequate financing for nursing education (Nutting, 1926). They also recommended that nursing schools should have separate governing boards, that students should work no more than 48 hours a week, that high school graduation should be required for admission, and that the objective of the system should be changed from a service to an educational one. If this were done, the period of training could be shortened to 28 months, and it would still furnish a better education than three years of service (Committee, 1923).

The second major effort to use the report strategy as a reform mechanism occurred in 1926 when the Committee on the Grading of Nursing Schools was set up. The Committee consisted of 21 persons from educational and health fields. Funds were supplied by a variety of donors, including the nursing organizations, foundations, individual nurses, and private philanthropists. Again the services of an outside researcher were secured; May Ayres Burgess, a statistician, directed the project. Although the Committee started with more modest goals, their work continued for eight years and included several significant reports. The first documented that there was widespread unemployment among nurses (Burgess, 1928).

Two waves of questionnaires were then sent out to the nursing schools in 1929 (Committee, 1930) and 1932 (Committee, 1932), the last at the height of the depression. The data were used to substantiate recommendations as well as to rate schools. The Committee urged that unaccredited and small hospitals with less than 50 beds close their schools. They argued that no school should continue to operate in a hospital that did not employ at least four registered nurses, including at least one instructor who was at least a high school graduate. They further recommended that the school should close if it worked its students more than eight hours a day or 56 hours a week, or expected them to carry head nurse and supervisory positions, or kept no records, or sent students out to do private duty nursing for the profit of the hospital (Committee, 1934).

The moral persuasion of the Committee was buttressed in this period by the serious unemployment situation. Some graduate nurses were so desperate that they were willing to work for board and room, or they were sent to work in hospitals with their wages paid by federal make-work projects (Rose, 1932; Schwitalla, 1933; Woodward, 1934). Under these circumstances, many small hospitals closed their schools. The number of schools fell from a high of 1885 in 1929 to 1781 in 1932 (Stewart, 1945, p. 209) and to 1311 in 1940 (Nursing Information Bureau, 1941).

In response to this series of reports and the unemployment situation, most states raised their requirements for the accreditation of schools. As a result, the era of the gross exploitation of student nurses began drawing to a close since most of the remaining schools met the minimum requirements of the grading committee. In 1949 Margaret West and Christy Hawkins surveyed nursing schools and found that the work weeks for student nurses had fallen from 54 hours in 1929 to 48 hours, while their class hours in the biological and behavorial sciences and in nursing had approximately doubled (West & Hawkins, 1950). In 1929 there had been 623 schools associated with hospitals with less than 50 beds, but by 1949 there were only 27 (West & Hawkins, 1950, p. 10).

Although these improvements seem modest by today's standards, the effect was to take most of the profit out of running a nursing school

(Kuhn, 1937). When this happened, the trend to close quickened. Since that time, costs have escalated so there are few hospitals that can afford the luxury of operating a school (Lysaught, 1974).

THE STRATIFICATION OF NURSING

As the struggle to raise educational standards progressed, nurses and hospital administrators decided all nursing tasks did not require a full three- or four-year education program. The solution was to stratify the role into two levels, registered professional and practical nursing. The first license for practical nurses was established in New York State in 1938, and the idea rapidly gained currency by the crisis in nursing brought on by World War II (Bullough & Bullough, 1978). By 1960 all of the states and territories had statutes licensing practical nurses (United States Department of Health, Education and Welfare, 1968).

The growing stratification of nursing made it easier to argue that the top strata needed university education. At the same time, both medical and nursing care were becoming more complex, so the need for better backgrounds in the biological and behavioral sciences was more apparent. Gradually more colleges and universities established collegiate programs. It was, however, a slow, uphill struggle, and it is only now that the collegiate schools have expanded sufficiently to take over a significant portion of nursing education. Consequently in the 1950s, the associate degree entry into academia opened up through the community colleges. This movement was pioneered by Mildred Montag. Her plan was well received and programs were established in New York, New Jersey, Michigan, Utah, California, and Virginia (Montag & Gotkin, 1959). Graduates of these programs demonstrated clinical competence equal to those of the hospital training school students and did as well on state board examinations (Montag, 1972), although it was necessary to modify some state regulations for them to be licensed. Increasingly this was done, and to further facilitate the growth of community college nursing education, the W. K. Kellogg Foundation in 1959 funded additional projects in California, New York, Texas, and Florida, which involved master's degree programs to prepare potential faculty members, continuing education sessions for faculty already in the field, the establishment of new associate degree nursing programs, and consultation whenever needed. By the time the project terminated five years later, more than 100 schools had been assisted (Anderson, 1966).

With this beginning the community college movement flourished. Growth was rapid. In 1962 students from associate degree

TABLE 1. BASIC NURSING PROGRAMS TO PREPARE
REGISTERED NURSES

Year	Diploma	Baccalaureate	Associate of Arts	Total
1873	5	—	—	5
1880	15	—	—	15
1890	35	—	—	35
1900	432	—	—	432
1910	1,129	—	—	1,129
1920	1,755	11	—	1,766
1930	1,885	23	—	1,908
1940	1,311	76	—	1,387[a]
1950	993	195	—	1,190[a]
1960	908	172	57	1,137[a]
1970	640	258	444	1,342[a]
1980	303	393	726	1,422

[a]Basic master's degree programs not included. *(Sources: M. A. Nutting. Educational status of nursing. United States Bureau of Education, Bulletin 1912, No. 7. Washington D.C.: U.S. Government Printing Office, 1912; Committee for the Study of Nursing and J. Goldmark. Nursing and nursing education in United States. New York: Macmillan, 1923; M. West and C. Hawkins. Nursing schools at mid-century. New York: National Committee for the Improvement of Nursing Service, 1950; Facts about nursing. American Nurses' Association, 1941, 1950, 1961, and 1970–1971 eds.; J. C. Vaughn. Educational preparation for nursing. Nursing and Health Care 3, October 1982, 447–455.)*

programs constituted 3.7% of the graduating registered nurses and by 1972 they constituted 37% of the graduating class, a tenfold increase in one decade. As Table 1 indicates, the associate degree programs replaced the hospital diploma programs as the basic mode of nursing education for bedside nurses.

CONTROVERSY OVER THE CAREER LADDER

Montag had argued that the associate degree should be a terminal degree because the objectives, content, and teaching methods of the community college were so different from the baccalaureate programs. She was strongly opposed to the "career ladder" concept of curriculum development where associate degree nurses could build on their community college experience by going to a baccalaureate school (Montag & Gotkin, 1959).

In line with this philosophy of two kinds of nurses instead of two levels, nursing educators conceptualized associate degree nurses as competent technicians who would work in concert with and under the supervision of physicians to move the patient toward recovery; i.e., they would give technical care. Baccalaureate-level nurses would be more independent practitioners, able to take a broader view of patient care, with an emphasis on the social and psychological problems of the patients (Rogers, 1961; Hassenplug, 1965; Johnson, 1966; Waters, et al., 1972). This would enable the better educated nurse, the baccalaureate nurse, to assume some of the bedside functions once relegated to the vocational nurses. Philosophically, the role was broken down in what has been called a care-cure dichotomy. The cure aspect, the more technical aspect that was under the control of the physician, would be given by the associate degree registered nurse, while the care aspect, a more independent role, would be the realm of the baccalaureate nurse. The major public document promulgating this point of view was a position paper published in 1965 by the Committee on Education of the American Nurses' Association (ANA, 1965).

This differentiation of roles was difficult to implement in the practice setting, particularly in the hospitals. Most hospital administrators regarded a registered nurse as a registered nurse. They were reluctant to differentiate functions or pay nurses with the baccalaureate degrees more money. They were willing to encourage nurses to give more psychological support to patients, but such support had to be done in conjunction with other nursing tasks, and they did not distinguish between the levels of educational preparation support.

Probably the major problem with the dichotomy was the fact that associate degree nurses never conceptualized themselves as a different kind of nurse, nor did they view their education as terminal. In a study reported in 1979, Bullough found that 75% of the associate degree students in a sample of 770 intended to continue their education to at least the level of a baccalaureate degree. In that same study, which included a total of 1,294 students from a consortium of seven Southern California nursing programs, no significant differences were found between associate degree and baccalaureate students in their orientation toward caring for or curing patients (Bullough, 1979).

Thus given the current situation in nursing, a career ladder option is apparently needed. Although generic baccalaureate programs continue their slow and steady growth, as shown in Table 1, the associate degree program is still the largest basic educational program, and a significant number of associate degree graduates want further education. Career ladder options were strongly recommended by the report of the National Commission on Nursing and Nursing Education directed by Jerome Lysaught. This report sponsored by private foundations, including the Kellogg Foundation, also strongly recommended that nursing education move out of the hospitals and into the mainstream of education in the colleges and universities (Lysaught, 1970).

The most recent large-scale study of nursing was sponsored by the American Hospital Association with support from private foundations. A group of 31 individuals, entitled the National Commission on Nursing, was recruited from hospital administration, nursing administration, nursing education, and a variety of organizations. The commissioners started an extensive literature review in 1980, then held a series of forums around the country. The final report, published in 1983, noted and supported the trend to upgrade nursing education, and the growth in graduate and baccalaureate programs, and urged private and governmental support of these programs. At the same time, the report supported the career ladder instead of urging a total baccalaureate work cadre. The paragraph summarizing several of the recommendations on education reads as follows:

> All types of nursing education programs, which continue to be needed, increasingly operating within the mainstream of higher education and in accordance with local circumstances and statewide planning, should hasten progress toward availability of baccalaureate and higher degrees for those desirous and capable of achieving them. Educational mobility and re-entry opportunities should be promoted within the educational system. Accreditation processes should respond to these needs and trends. (National Commission on Nursing, 1983)

THE BACCALAUREATE ENTRY INTO PROFESSIONAL PRACTICE PROPOSAL

In spite of this recommendation, there is a substantial group within nursing that would like to see one educational pattern for all registered nurses and a different one for practical nurses. The vehicle for enforcing this approach would be the state nurse practice acts. The movement started in New York State in 1974, when the State Nurses' Association passed a resolution calling for the baccalaureate degree as the minimum preparation for entry into professional practice by 1985 (New York State Nurses' Association, 1974). This resolution quickly became the focus of a national discussion, and in 1976 the Council of Baccalaureate and Higher Degrees of the National League for Nursing (NLN) passed a similar resolution. The idea gained further support when a package of three entry-into-practice resolutions were passed by the American Nurses' Association (ANA, 1978). Subsequently, various other nursing organizations have debated the issue and some, including most notably the Association of Operating Room

Nurses, have supported the movement. In 1982 the Board of Directors of the National League for Nursing (representing all of the Councils: Practical, Associate Degree, Diploma, and Baccalaureate)

The resolutions are emerging as one of the major issues facing the profession today, although there are differences of opinion as to what the resolutions mean, whether or not they should be implemented, and what their implementation would do for the profession.

DIFFERING VIEWS OF THE ENTRY-INTO-PRACTICE RESOLUTIONS

It seems clear that the New York State Nurses' Association did not have a career ladder in mind when it passed the original resolution. Rather, the Association seemed to have conceptualized the baccalaureate graduate as the registered nurse, whereas nurses with associate degrees were to be technical or practical nurses. Articulation between the two groups of nurses was not spelled out in the original resolution, although there was considerable sentiment in favor of some type of grandfather clause that would allow existing registered nurses the right to retain their current titles.

The 1978 ANA resolutions were quite different in focus from the original New York proposal. They clearly called for increased accessibility to high-quality career mobility programs, using flexible approaches for individuals seeking academic degrees in nursing. Thus, they deal with the problem of the existing work force by advocating continued education rather than the grandfather clause.

The 1982 resolutions by the NLN Board of Directors were made with career ladder opportunities in mind. This support for educational mobility is a function of time and a growing political sophistication among nurses. Serious attempts to turn the resolutions into laws have taken place only in New York and Ohio. The Ohio Nurses' Association has delayed basic reform of the nurse practice act to cover current levels of practice, in order to link that reform with a proposal to make the baccalaureate degree a requirement for the registered nurse level. In New York, the proposal in the form of a bill has been introduced in every legislative session since 1975. Although it has had the devoted support of several legislators, the bill has never been voted out of committee. Legislators are afraid to support it because they receive a storm of protest whenever it is considered seriously. One reason for this is that as late as 1975, 80% of the nursing work force in New York were diploma or associate degree graduates. Many saw the proposal as denigrating their nursing preparation and squeezing them out of the job market. They were particularly angry when the proposal was linked with an anticareer ladder stance.

The New York State Nurses' Association has now moved to a procareer ladder stance, but the legislature is cautious about backing any nursing legislation because of the bitter infighting they saw among nurses. It will take a long process of image building to reestablish the Nurses' Association credibility. Meanwhile, other state associations have watched the New York experience and have reacted with caution.

When the issue is examined on its merits, there are arguments that can be made both for and against the proposal. Supporters of the idea see it as a means of bringing order into a disorderly educational system. They look at the system described above and point out that patients, the public, and colleagues within the health care delivery team would be less confused if we settled on one standard program for the preparation of registered nurses. Advocates look at the growing complexity of patient care and know that nurses need more education, both in the biological and behavioral sciences, as well as in clinical nursing. Moving into the university should improve the knowledge base and enable nurses to give better patient care. University graduation will also "professionalize" the occupation, which will give nurses more status and more power over patient care decisions. These are potent arguments in favor of the resolutions (Christy, 1980; Lynaugh, 1980; Partridge, 1981).

Opponents of the proposal do not perceive the baccalaureate degree as needed for all nursing functions. Some do not even believe that current baccalaureate programs are the best educational preparation for nursing. The American Hospital Association is against the proposal simply because there are not enough existing baccalaureate graduates to staff the nation's hospitals. With a grandfather clause, the existing staffing could continue, but since few legislatures will seriously consider such a clause, the proposal if passed into law could cause a crisis in the hospitals.

GRADUATE EDUCATION

As nursing moves into the colleges and universities at both the associate degree and baccalaureate levels, another problem emerges. The movement into colleges and community colleges forced nurses to upgrade their education because to be successful in colleges, nurses needed the same kind of academic credentials that their colleagues in other departments had. At first they did not have this and as late as 1953, a survey found that only 36% of the faculty in college programs had earned a master's degree. Most, 51%, were at the bachelor-degree level, while 13% had no degree at all (Bullough & Bullough, 1978, p. 198). Nurses sought to remedy their deficiency, but as they went on to graduate school or attempted to enter graduate school, they found themselves at a tremendous disadvantage. Graduate education for the most part is specialty education, and persons are trained to be sociologists, historians, psychologists, anatomists, by other sociologists, historians, psychologists, anatomists, and there is a general assumption that people getting these degrees had undergraduate majors or at least a strong minor in them. This meant that nurses who wanted to go on for graduate study after receiving a baccalaureate in nursing had to establish themselves in another field of study. This was difficult to do in any field but probably was easiest in education where nursing already had established ties with such institutions as Teachers College. In fact, Teachers College had started accepting graduates with nursing baccalaureate into its master's degree programs almost as soon as nurses began to earn bachelor's degrees. Other universities such as Chicago, which opened a special graduate program to prepare nursing administrators and teachers, did so in conjunction with the School of Education. Inevitably, most nurses who went on for advanced study did so in education, and nursing faculties came to be dominated by people who had earned a higher degree in education.

It was not only because educational programs threw less obstacles in the path of nurses that they were so attractive, but also because many schools of education were accustomed to part-time graduate students since many of their programs were designed for teachers or administrators who attended after the school day was over. Many of the more traditional degree programs discouraged the part-time student. Still another reason that nurses went to schools of education was because they were women, and the field of education discriminated less against women than almost any other graduate area of study. As early as 1900, more women earned doctorates in education than any other field, and education continued to be far more receptive to the female candidate than other disciplines.

Few nurses went beyond a master's degree in education until nursing itself began offering graduate work. Even as late as 1950, only an estimated 28 nurses had even obtained a doctorate in any field. The number slowly began increasing after that until by 1970, 535 nurses had obtained doctorates, although degrees in education continued to outnumber those in all other fields (Bullough & Bullough, 1978, pp. 198–199). Education degrees helped form some of the ways in which nursing developed. Education programs traditionally have not demanded the research component present in other doctoral programs, if only because education itself suffered from some of the same disadvantages that nursing did, in comparison with graduate programs in the liberal arts or in the other professions. Teacher education had been carried out mainly in the normal schools, many of which had been equivalent to high schools. Gradually the level of teacher education was raised in this country, but in states like Ohio it was only in the 1950s that normal school degrees were no longer recognized. Thus education in many of the graduate schools in the country was struggling to upgrade itself, just as nurses were trying to do for themselves. In a way, the nursing reliance on professional education was an example of the blind leading the halt, and although nursing and education helped each other in raising standards, education (and nursing) never quite achieved the respectability in most graduate schools that other disciplines did.

When the nurse graduates of these programs went out to teach other nurses, they found themselves at a further disadvantage compared with other academic disciplines in the college, in that they held advanced degrees in areas other than the ones in which they were teaching. Most of their graduate work had concentrated on educational rather than nursing material, although some graduate schools had offered courses geared to nursing education. For the most part, however, graduate degrees in education were aimed at either those planning to teach education in college or those who were teaching or administering at the elementary and secondary level. Thus there was an emphasis on curriculum, supervision, social foundations of education, educational psychology, or some similar field that indirectly might have had some bearing on nursing but that did not concentrate on research techniques or on specific nursing problems. When these new doctorates were hired as nursing faculty, they tried to implement what they had learned in their graduate course work. Carol J. Willts Peterson claimed that nurse educators were so involved in adopting new trends and themes in curriculum and instruction, they had little time to think about the trends in nursing. Moreover, they were so zealous in perpetuating the ideology of the educational schools, their innovations lost all flexibility and instead became structural barriers that upheld a continuing rigid system of education (Peterson, 1983, p. 95).

Peterson's survey of nursing education was highly critical, but the things she found are common to all schools of education. For example, Peterson stated that nursing programs seem to be obsessed with curriculum revisions. Curricula are constantly being revised, and nursing educators inevitably see a problem in nursing as being solvable by a revision in their curriculum. As a result, funding for large-scale curriculum revision is always being sought, curriculum revision coordinators are named, and deans and directors seek extra funds to release faculty to work on curriculum matters. One result of this is that nursing, at least in the immediate past, rather than doing research on basic issues affecting nursing, has spent much of its time in studying or implementing curriculum revision. Since curriculum, however, is a major study area for those getting degrees in education, it seems that this is an inevitable consequence of the kind of training that nurses have received.

Peterson also reported that nursing educators put more emphasis on behavioral objectives in teaching than any other areas in the college except schools of education. Faculty members, in her words, "write objectives until the finiteness of the statements borderlines on the ridiculous. Tests are blueprinted religiously according to objectives and items coded according to objectives and cognitive level." An inevitable result of such rigid implementation of a valued educational technique is a fractionalized view of nursing, coupled with an unwillingness on behalf of many nursing students to read on their own for content, unless the objectives are clearly outlined. Rote memorization is encouraged with a compilation of lists of five principles of this and seven principles of that, instead of trying to encourage nursing students to examine basic problems themselves. Such techniques are probably very good for the teacher doing fifth-grade teaching, but not necessarily for collegiate-level nurses who ultimately deal with life-and-death matters.

As schools of education moved in the last few decades to develop new teaching modalities, their nurse graduates religiously brought these methods to the nursing schools. The tremendous involvement of nursing instructors in individualized, modular, self-paced instruction forces them to turn out massive syllabi designed to aid the student. The result is to make the teacher almost extraneous. Inevitably, nursing schools have become the most conspicuous users of photo-copying machines and mimeographs, and nursing syllabi not only fill the shelves of the college bookstores, but nurses either intentionally or unintentionally are large-scale violators of copyright laws. One serious consequence of this is that teachers tend to spend so much of their time keeping their syllabi updated that they cannot do the necessary research to get promoted in the university setting, even though person for person they probably work harder at their teaching than faculty members in almost any other discipline. Underlying this nursing commitment to individualized, modular, self-paced instruction is some basic research in competency-based instruction and mastery development, but nursing educators are so immersed in the movement, their methodology so structured and cumbersome, that the potential benefit of some of the technologies has been lost.

It is the history of nursing education that sets the issues for today. It seems clear that if nursing had not established the associate degree, it might be easier to require a baccalaureate degree since there would have been no alternative to the decrease in diploma schools. Alternatively, if with the development of the associate degrees the baccalaureate nurses had emphasized the development of nursing specialty, there would have been a clear demarcation between the two levels of nurses, and perhaps the baccalaureate entry level could be justified. But realistically it was the success of the associate degree that weakened the diploma programs, and without them, nursing would have been hard pressed to meet the demand for nurses. Politically, because of the expansion of the graduate programs into nursing specialties and away from nursing education, it becomes possible to distinguish between master-level-prepared nurses and the R.N., but nursing itself, or at least organized nursing, has not yet come to terms with this kind of distinction. We predict that this, and not the resolution on baccalaureate nursing, will be the growing issue of the 1980s. The growth of nursing specialties will also change the nature of nursing education, encouraging the development of Ph.D. or Doctorates of Nursing in nursing subjects. It is hoped that by 1990 the nursing doctorates will be numerous enough that nurses need not take doctorates in other fields. Then, and only then, will nursing have finally made it as an academic discipline on a par with others in the colleges and universities.

REFERENCES

American Nurses' Association Convention, '78. *American Journal of Nursing,* July, 1978, pp. 1230–1246.

American Nurses' Association. First position paper on education for nursing. *American Journal of Nursing,* December 1965, pp. 106–111.

Anderson, B. E. *Nursing education in community junior colleges.* Philadelphia: Lippincott, 1966.

Bullough, B. The associate degree: Beginning or end? *Nursing Outlook,* 1979, **27,** 324–328.

Bullough, V. L. & Bullough, B. *Care of the sick: The emergence of modern nursing.* New York: Prodist, Neale Watson, 1978.

Burgess, M. A. *Nurses, patients and pocketbooks.* New York: Committee on the Grading of Nursing Schools, 1928.

Christy, T. *Cornerstone for nursing education: A history of the division of nursing education of Teachers College, Columbia University, 1899–1947.* New York: Teachers College Press, 1969.

Christy, T. Entry into practice: A recurring issue in nursing history. *American Journal of Nursing,* March 1980, pp. 485–488.

Committee for the Study of Nursing Education, J. Goldmark, Sec. *Nursing and nursing education in the United States.* New York: Macmillian, 1923.

Committee on the Grading of Nursing Schools. *Results of the first grading study in nursing schools.* New York: Macmillian, 1930.

Committee on the Grading of Nursing Schools. *The second grading of nursing schools.* New York: Macmillian, 1932.

Committee on the Grading of Nursing Schools. *Nursing schools today and tomorrow: Final report.* New York: Macmillian, 1934, pp. 197–213.

Cunningham, E. V. Education for leadership in nursing 1899–1959. *Nursing Outlook,* May 1959, pp. 268–272.

Flexner, A. *Medical education in the United States and Canada.* New York: Carnegie Foundation, 1910.

Gray, J. *Education for nursing: History of the University of Minnesota school of nursing.* Minneapolis: University of Minnesota, 1960.

Hassenplug, L. Preparation of the nurse practitioner. *Journal of Nursing Education,* 1965, **4,** 29–42.

Hintz, A. A. The probationary term. In J. Hodson (Ed.), *How to become a trained nurse.* New York: Abbatt, 1898, pp. 15–19.

Hintz, A. A. The training term. In J. Hodson (Ed.), *op. cit.,* pp. 20–24.

Hodson, J. (Ed.). *How to become a trained nurse.* New York: Abbatt, 1898, p. 256; pp. 110–227.

Jamme, A. C. The California eight-hour law for women. *American Journal of Nursing,* April 1919, 525–530.

Johnson, D. Competence in practice: technical and professional. *Nursing Outlook,* 1966, **14,** 30–33.

Kuhn, J. K. Financial demands of the new curriculum on the school of nursing. *Hospital Management,* December 1937, pp. 41–43.

Lynaugh, J. P. The entry into practice conflict: How we got where we are and what will happen next. *American Journal of Nursing,* February 1980, pp. 266–270.

Lysaught, J. P. *An abstract for action.* New York: McGraw-Hill, 1970.

Lysaught, J. P. Costs of nursing education and a case for its greater support. In J. P. Lysaught (Ed.), *Action in nursing: Progress in professional purpose.* New York: McGraw-Hill, 1974.

MacDonald, G. *Development of standards and accreditation in collegiate nursing education.* New York: Teachers College Press, 1965, p. 53.

Montag, M. *Evaluation of graduates of associate degree nursing programs.* New York: Teachers College Press, 1972.

Montag, M. & Gotkin, L. G. *Community college education for nursing.* New York: McGraw-Hill, 1959.

Munson, H. W. & Stevens, K. *The story of the National League of Nursing Education.* Philadelphia: Saunders, 1934.

National Commission on Nursing. *Summary Report and Recommendations.* Chicago: Hospital Research and Educational Trust, 1983.

National League for Nursing. *Criteria for the appraisal of baccalaureate and higher degree programs in nursing.* 5th ed. New York: National League for Nursing, 1983.

National League of Nursing Education. *Curriculum for schools of nursing.* New York: NLNE, 1927.

National League of Nursing Education. *Curriculum guide for schools of nursing.* New York: NLNE, 1937.

New York State Nurses' Association. *Resolution on entry into professional practice.* Albany: The Association, 1974.

Nursing Information Bureau of the American Nurses' Association. *Facts about nursing.* New York: ANA, 1941, p. 21.

Nutting, M. A. *A sound economic basis for schools of nursing and other addresses.* New York: Putnam, 1926, pp. 3–17.

Nutting, M. A. & Dock, L. L. *A history of nursing, Vol. II.* New York: Putnam, 1907, pp. 388–393.

Partridge, R. Education for entry into professional nursing practice: The planning of change. *Journal of Nursing Education,* 1981, **20,** 40–46.

Peterson, C. J. W. Overview of issues in nursing education. In N. L. Chaska (Ed.), *The nursing profession: A time to speak.* New York: McGraw-Hill, 1983, pp. 91–99.

Richards, L. Recollections of a pioneer nurse. *American Journal of Nursing,* January 1903, pp. 245–252.

Richards, L. Early days in the first American training school for nurses. *American Journal of Nursing,* September 1973, pp. 574–575.

Rogers, M. *Educational revolution in nursing.* New York: Macmillan, 1961.

Rose, M. L. What about our own catastrophe. *American Journal of Nursing,* January 1932, pp. 62–63.

Schwitalla, A. M. Present economic objectives of the nursing profession. *American Journal of Nursing,* December 1933, pp. 1135–1142.

Standard Curriculum for Schools of Nursing. New York: National League of Nursing Education, 1917.

Stewart, I. M. The movement for shorter hours in nurses' training schools. *American Journal of Nursing,* March 1919, pp. 439–443.

Stewart, I. M. *The education of nurses: Historical foundations and modern trends.* New York: Macmillan, 1945, p. 106.

United States Department of Health, Education and Welfare. *State licensing of health occupations.* Public Health Service Pub. No. 1758. Washington, D. C.: U. S. Government Printing Office, 1968, pp. 9–10.

Waters, V., Chater, S., Vivier, M. L., et al. Technical and professional nursing: An exploratory study. *Nursing Research* March–April 1972, **21,** 124–131.

West, M. & Hawkins, C. *Nursing schools at the mid-century.* New York: National Committee for the Improvement of Nursing Services, 1950, pp. 10; 52–53.

Woodham-Smith, C. *Florence Nightingale 1820–1910.* New York: McGraw-Hill, 1951, pp. 233–238; 352.

Woodward, E.S. Federal aspects of unemployment among professional women. *American Journal of Nursing,* June 1934, pp. 534–538.

CHAPTER 6

Theory in Nursing

The function of theory is to impose order on what might appear to be chaos, and it does so by being in some measure abstract. In this sense, religious explanations of the universe and the place of men and women in the world are theories. They are, however, usually not scientific theories since the essential difference between a scientific theory and a religious one is that a scientific theory is predictable. If a stone is dropped from a tower, we can predict that it will drop to the ground because it follows the theory of gravity. When theories, such as gravity, have become accepted as basic rules, they then are recognized as laws.

Theory as we know it today was originally developed by the ancient Greeks, and ancient Greek ideas about the nature of the universe, the causes of disease, the ideal government, and various other areas we today label as the sciences, the social sciences, and the humanities, have had great influence on our cultural mindset. The Greeks were among the first people to try to explain the world and its workings in a natural way, instead of relying on supernatural explanations.

It was the Greeks, for example, who advanced the geocentric theory of the universe, that the earth was the center of the universe. They did not pull this theory out of thin air, but after considering various alternative assumptions, including the heliocentric one, they found that only the geocentric universe answered all the questions. But knowledge does not remain static and as advances in knowledge and understanding took place, the geocentric theory became ever more elaborate. It also became part of religion since religion tends to incorporate scientific explanations into its own framework over time.

St. Thomas Aquinas in the thirteenth century used the geocentric theory to explain Christian dogma in a rational way. Christianity, he believed, was a logical and rational religion, and it was important to him that science and religion agree in those areas where there was knowable knowledge and observable phenomenon.

The incorporation of the geocentric theory into Christianity encouraged further experimentation and seeking of knowledge, and this in itself led to a basic challenge. For example, as astronomical observations became ever more sophisticated, it became evident that the moon and planets behaved in ways that could not easily be explained by assuming that all these bodies revolved in circles around the earth. Rather than discarding the theory, however, the old theory was patched up and modified to fit the newly discovered data and became ever more complicated. Although Nicholas Copernicus in the sixteenth century speculated that it was equally possible for the earth to move around the sun, the available data did not necessarily support his theory any better than the geocentric theory, and it left many questions unanswered such as why things fall to earth. The Greeks had answered this by saying that earth, which is the densest material, is at the center; everything made of such material tries to go to its natural place in the universe, i.e., to the center. Similarly, they argued that above the earth was the sphere of air and beyond that the sphere of fire, and so things made of air would float upward and fire as it burned would burn upward, both trying to find their natural place in the universe.

It was only after the telescope had been invented in the seventeenth century and Galileo could observe planets more accurately that so many more contradictions appeared in the geocentric theory that the heliocentric theory gained momentum. The final element in the victory of the new heliocentric theory was the concept of gravity as developed by Sir Isaac Newton. Ultimately the heliocentric theory won because it could not only explain things well but could do so in much simpler terms. In general, in science when a simple theory can explain everything as well as a complex one, scientists opt for the more simple explanation. The result of the discoveries of Copernicus and Newton has been called the scientific revolution (Bullough, 1970; Kuhn, 1962).

Theories are not devised for their own sake. There is a process involved in which the observable facts and experimental data are gathered together, and then this more or less random information is put into some kind of order. In philosophical terms, we have established a paradigm, a model of reality that can then channel and direct other experimental or exploratory data. A good example of a theory that is still subject to some controversy, at least among the nonscientific community, is Darwin's theory of evolution. During the past decade, a group of people known as creationists have argued that the theory of evolution is just one possible explanation of how life developed, and that there are equally attractive alternatives. Although the creationists are mostly biblical literalists, they argue that their theory is not adopted for religious but for scientific reasons. No scientific data, however, support the creationists, whereas every aspect of science from geology to biology to microbiology to biochemistry supports the concept of evolution.

A more controversial well-known theory is that of Karl Marx's dialectical materialism. Some societies, such as the Soviet Union, regard Marx's theory as dogma, not subject to empirical verification. Many Americans who call themselves Marxists see a great deal of truth in Marx's theory, particularly in his emphasis on the needs of men and women for material things such as food and shelter as a key to understanding the organization of society, although they would not in any sense of the word be regarded as Soviet Communists. The difficulty with Marxist theory, however, is that much of it remains untestable. For this reason there is much more disagreement about it, as well as about other economic and social theories, than there is about scientific theories.

Theories, however, like religion, serve still another purpose, and it is probably for this reason that there are so many theory makers. Theories both chart courses of action for practitioners and make it possible to develop impressive rationales for action. Historically, medicine and the health sciences have proved to be particularly susceptible to grand theories. A major reason for this is that the practitioners, usually physicians, knew so little but claimed so much. The only way such claims could be accepted was by a kind of self- or group-validation. This was easier to do in medicine than in many other areas because of what we know as the "placebo effect." This also encouraged the rise of conflicting theories. But the health professionals also worked under a handicap, because if a patient came to them, and the specialists said that they did not know the answer, the person would just go elsewhere until someone could identify the cause of the illness. By erecting theories, the health professional could give an answer to every question and a solution to every problem. Many patients got better with or without the activities of the practitioner, so the medical theories appeared valid, at least part of the time.

The Greeks contributed several medical theories, but the dominant one was the humoral explanation of illness found in the Hippocratic corpus and popularized by Galen in the second century A.D.

The Hippocratic writers, following the theory of a geocentric universe, regarded the body as made up of the same four elements that made up the universe: earth, water, air, and fire. Each of these elements had its particular quality: cold, hot, dry, wet, and the nature of the body was determined by physical representatives of these elements: blood, phlegm, yellow bile, and black bile. When each of these elements existed in the correct proportion, the body was healthy; pain resulted or illness came about when one of them was found either deficient or excessive. Blood came from the heart and represented heat; phlegm came from the brain and represented cold; yellow bile, which represented dryness, was secreted by the liver, whereas black bile, derived from the spleen and liver, symbolized wetness.

There were various modifications of the theory but most of the ancient physicians assumed, as do the modern advocates of holistic medicine, that wellness was the natural state of being, and only when something intervened to prevent this or disturb the humoral distribution did sickness, pain, and death result. As in the geocentric theory, elaboration of the theory developed with the anatomical discoveries of the late Middle Ages and Harvey's discovery of the circulation of the blood in the seventeenth century. No physician worth his salt would admit to not being able to give a theoretical reason for illness. (There were no women physicians in the seventeenth century.) Some of the theories demanded strenuous intervention such as bloodletting, starvation, and purging, which in themselves frequently proved more dangerous than the illness. Each theoretical school tried to develop unified theoretical frameworks. Thus the group that conceptualized illness as caused by hypertension used phlebotomy to treat a wide range of symptoms, including what we now call anemia. When their patients complained that the medical remedies were killing them, physicians used their theories to explain why this could not be so and why, as physicians, they were right. One result of such strong medical intervention was a hostility to formalized medical practitioners in the eighteenth and nineteenth centuries and a turn to nontraditional practitioners. Historians who study past medical theories often ask themselves when the physician or surgeon, the two key medical professionals, really began to help people more than handicap them, to cure them instead of killing them. The answer usually given is about the beginning of the twentieth century.

In fact it was only toward the end of the nineteenth century, as a consequence of the discovery of bacteria, that we could really begin to explain what caused most illnesses. Almost immediately we could begin to deal with causal factors and find vaccines, antidotes, and other weapons to deal with illness. This broke down the grand theories because different causes were identified for each illness. As this happened, various theory makers in medicine began to come together. The alleopaths and homeopaths and various other schools of theory merged to become the modern physician. One group, the osteopaths, remained outside of the organized medical community for a longer time, insisting on some special techniques, including manipulation, but adopting the germ theory as well. Chiropractors were more rigid in their theory and it took longer for them to accept the discoveries and begin to move into the mainstream. Still there is considerable room in medicine for advocates of a special theory, such as chiropractors, because there is still much about the functions of the human body we do not know. The more we know, however, the less valid the theorists become. Our knowledge is greatest in the physical aspects of the human body, less so in terms of the psychosocial aspect of illness. Thus psychiatry as well as psychiatric nursing has many different modes of treatment, depending on whose theory a particular physician or nurse is following. Increasingly, however, the domain of speculation is lessened as behavioral and biological science advance, and we learn more about the chemical factors underlying certain forms of mental illness.

Interestingly, the more we know about certain areas of medicine, the more likely we are to posit theories about areas we do not know and to widen what becomes a medical problem to take in more and more territory. This is particularly notable in the field of pediatrics, which found itself increasingly concerned with well babies and children as we successfully lessened the dangers of childhood diseases. Being a pediatrician was not as challenging as it once had been, and so pediatricians elaborated new theories to expand their scope of practice. Children today are treated not only for their physical conditions, most of them minor, but for an expanding list of behavioral, emotional, and social problems that include poor school performance, hyperactivity, shyness, aggressive and antisocial behavior, resistance to discipline, compulsive behavior, temper tantrum, and peer rejection (Burnett & Bell, 1978; Haggert & Janeway, 1960). Many of these behaviors were conceptualized in the past in nonmedical terms and subject to forms of social control rather than medical treatment. Depending on the age of the child and the nature and severity of the problem, control might have taken the form of school or parental discipline, or the supervision of juvenile authorities. Today, children who exhibit such behaviors are regarded as legitimate concerns for the medical profession. Because we know less about the reasons for these behaviors than we do about bacterial infections, we are freer to speculate, to hypothesize, and to make theories, and so theory making in these areas has become all important. Apparently, if pediatricians are any example, we love to theorize about that which we do not know.

NURSING THEORY

In a recent work on theory construction, Walker and Avant (1983) identify four levels of theory development in nursing:

1. Meta theory development,
2. Grand theory development,
3. Middle range theory, and
4. Practice theory.

The meta theory level is theory about theories. Examples of meta theory in nursing would be the various theory conferences that have been held in the past two decades, or more recently, in works analyzing theories (Norris, 1969; Norris, 1970; Norris, 1971; The Nursing Development Conference Group, 1973; Chinn, 1983). Most of the well-known theory building has been at the grand theory level. Theory building at the middle range and the practice theory level is fairly common but less well recognized.

Grand theory in nursing tends to be aimed at conceptualizing a generalized prescription for nursing actions or a generalized work role. These theories tend to include the following three elements:

1. An assumption about the range of patient problems that nurses address. This statement often breaks down the task of delivering health care and assigns portions of the work to nurses, physicians, and others. Usually the nursing role includes the whole nursing team.
2. An assumption about the nature of illness or patient and client problems.
3. Given these two assumptions, a therapeutic nursing approach is outlined.

Historically, the first nursing theorist was probably Florence Nightingale, who emphasized the environment of the sick person as all important. She viewed disease as a reparative process, an effort to remedy a previous process of "poisoning and decay." Nurses were all-important in this because health could be restored by the "proper use of fresh air, warmth, cleanliness, quiet, and the proper selection and administration of diet" (Nightingale, 1860). Nightingale assigned an active intervention role to surgeons and physicians. Their duty was to cut out an offending organ or otherwise intervene in the disease process. To nurses she assigned the more indirect role. She believed that nursing's primary duty was to "put the patient in the best condition for nature to act uppn him" (Nightingale, 1860). She felt that women were particularly well-suited to this supportive role and fought to establish nursing as a woman's profession.

Nightingale, however, was writing at a time before the bacterial revolution had taken place, and although the environment of the sick person remained a key concept of nursing, the idea was modified to include measures designed to avoid the spread of infection, to ease the patient's suffering, and to establish patient well-being. One of the major difficulties, however, is that nurses, except those in Catholic religious orders, were rarely consulted in the design and building of hospitals, and so their role in handling the environment was tempered by harsh reality. They had to make do with the buildings in which they found themselves, and many of these did not offer the patient a particularly cheerful environment. Similarly, as the hospital movement developed in United States in the twentieth century, physicians moved in to supervise diets, activity, and other nursing measures so that nursing decision making as Nightingale had conceptualized it was limited.

Such was the charisma of Nightingale that her definition of nursing was not challenged until well into the twentieth century, and it remains the key element in most contemporary theories of nursing. Without upsetting Nightingale's basic formulations, Bertha Harmer suggested that patient teaching and the education of younger nurses were important nursing functions (Nursing Development Conference Group, 1973; Harmer, 1922).

The genesis of serious consideration of the nursing role in the twentieth century started with scholars who were not nurses. Esther Lucille Brown, an anthropologist, studied nursing and reported her findings in *Nursing for the Future* (Brown, 1948).

Brown postulated that nurses of the future would be required to assume more supervisory and administrative duties, act as physicians' assistants, and assume more responsibility for preventive medicine. If nurses were to fulfill this expanded role, she felt that they should not waste their time and energy on activities that other less-skilled workers could do. Her report therefore recommended that auxiliary personnel, particularly practical nurses, be trained to work with the nursing team and that the professional nurse be used for the specialized nursing of the acutely ill, for supervision, for administering institutional nursing services, and for assisting the physician; professional nurses should do the planning, administration, and supervision within the community health services, teach health, and undertake the administration, teaching, and research within the schools of nursing (Brown, 1948).

In the 1950s the nursing role was analyzed by several sociologists. Lyle Saunders looked at nursing as an occupation that was highly diversified, isolated, and conservative. He saw nursing's responsibilities as complex, demanding advanced knowledge from many fields, yet the level of decision-making power was low. Like Brown, he predicted that nurses would be taking on more managerial responsibilities (Saunders, 1954).

In his analysis of the role of hospital nurses, Hans Mauksch also noted the complex role that nurses fill, with responsibilities for direct care as well as organizing and coordinating the care given by others. Both these responsibilities are made more complex by the dual hierarchy of the hospital, with physicians in charge of the clinical treatment of patients and hospital management in charge of administering the hospital work force. Nurses, especially head nurses, carried heavy responsibility for coordinating these two systems (Mauksch, 1957). A similar picture of the difficult role of nurses in the dual hierarchy of the hospital was presented by Smith (Smith, 1958).

Sociologists who studied nursing were not trying to build a generalized theory, yet sociology played a role in fostering nursing theory by providing basic concepts about the nursing role. In addition, sociologists furnished nursing with a variety of definitions of professions and analyses of the professionalization process, and most of these definitions included a theory base as an attribute of a profession. Nurses consciously decided to design and test theory in order to professionalize (Walker & Avant, 1983). The sociological studies of nursing also motivated nurses to analyze their own role instead of leaving the task to others. At first this tended to be mere task analysis.

This was seen as inadequate by many nursing educators because in their mind such studies did not contribute to the understanding of nursing practice, and so there was a shift from a focus on the total nursing role to a focus on direct patient care and the nature and purpose of the nurse-client relationship (Newman, 1983). Hildegard Peplau was important in this transition because she imported the interpersonal theories from psychiatry to nursing and provided a basis for nurses to begin to analyze the process of their interaction with patients in terms of its therapeutic qualities (Peplau, 1952). Other nurses turned to other disciplines for ideas and concepts. Ida Orlando utilized communication theory to describe what she termed "a deliberative nursing approach." She called it deliberative because she argued that an assessment phase should come before action. This was an important step in the development of the nursing process (Orlando, 1961). Imogene King explained the transactional processes occurring between nurse and patient (King, 1971).

One of the things that some of the nurse theoreticians did was to try to differentiate the nature of nursing practice from that of medical practice. One frequently cited definition of nursing was by Virginia Henderson, who indicated that nurses do for the patients what they cannot do for themselves, with the intent of promoting independence (Henderson, 1966). Dorothea Orem's approach to nursing was similar to that of Henderson. She argued that nursing services are needed by persons who are unable to take care of themselves because of health or health-related reasons. She saw this replacement of self-care as the special domain of nursing (Orem, 1971).

Sociological concepts were also utilized in this effort to differentiate medicine and nursing. Skipper had used the sociological terms *expressive* and *instrumental* to study nurses. Nurses with instrumental orientations were described as being concerned with getting the patient well, while the expressively oriented nurses were said to be focused more on the social and emotional problems. Skipper interviewed a sample of nursing students and registered nurses in one large metropolitan hospital and found most nurses had an expressive orientation (Skipper, 1965). Johnson and Martin (1965) then argued that the instrumental role was a medical role, while the expressive role was primarily a nursing role. Dorothy Johnson (1959) used this dichotomy as one of the basic assumptions in her early theory development. Having assigned the instrumental or curing role to medicine, she turned her analytical efforts to the caring aspects of health care delivery. Sister Callista Roy (1970), a student of Johnson, also accepted the differentiation and focused on the role of nursing as facilitating the adaptive potential of patients. Frances Kreuter (1957) felt that a focus on the care aspect of the nursing role was an important step in humanizing nursing services.

PATTERNING

Martha Rogers's theory development was at a little later date, so she was able to build on the earlier work in the field. She spent less time differentiating nursing and medicine but accepted the separation of focus as an assumption and turned her attention to describing the clients that nurses serve. She utilized the term *pattern* to describe human and environmental characteristics or a human process. She stated that "a concept of patterning incorporates within it recognition that it is the totality of the constituents that compose the pattern." Human and environmental patterns are dynamic, constantly changing, and the resulting pattern derives from the mutual interaction and mutual change (Rogers, 1970).

Nursing theory did not remain static. Rogers, for example, revised her terms to clarify concepts and to meet the concerns of her critics. In her early writing, the term patterns had covered the individual, the environment, and the interaction between them. In her later work, the term patterns was used only for the functioning of the individual and the environment, whereas the term *energy fields* was used to describe the interaction (Rogers, 1980).

Dorothy Johnson conceived of *patterns of functioning* as the repetitive and regular ways in which persons, in a stable state, meet their bodily needs and interpersonal needs (Johnson, 1961). For Johnson, illness disrupted an individual's usual patterns of functioning, creating a disequilibrium. The purpose of nursing was to help the patient find patterns of functioning that were maximally gratifying. This new equilibrium provided a degree of constancy in the patterns of functioning for the patient, both internally and interpersonally. She later used the term *set* to describe an individual's predisposition to act in certain ways rather than others. Individuals develop and use preferred ways of behaving under certain conditions (Johnson, 1980).

GRAND THEORY

There are another group of nursing theorists who have adapted their models from general systems theory. Betty Neuman is probably the most well-known of this group. She attempts to analyze all the needs of clients, their families, and communities in relationship to the stressors that cause them problems, and to identify the functions of nurses using the nursing process to solve those problems. Indirect nursing care is addressed as well as direct one-to-one care (Neuman, 1982).

Although the Neuman model is perhaps the grandest of all the theories mentioned above, all could be classified as grand theories. That is, they attempt to explain all or a major portion of nursing actions. Grand theories tend to be difficult to test. Consequently, nursing grand theories have tended to be used as a basis for practice or for curriculum building, but they have generated few hypotheses that have been tested in a systematic scientific process.

In spite of the profession's close relationship to sociology, nursing has not yet followed the path of sociology in withdrawing from general theorizing to move to theories of the middle range. The movement in sociology was led in part by Robert K. Merton, who argued eloquently that broad global concepts such as social systems, social institutions, social milieux, and values are not the areas where sociologists should direct their attention. Instead, he advocated "conceptual parsimony" as in the development of a paradigm that employs "the minimum set of concepts with which the sociologist must operate in order to carry through an adequate functional analysis" (Merton, 1957). Merton sought to formulate theoretically significant yet empirically testable hypotheses of sociological importance. Problem finding must occur, generally, before scientific solutions may be examined. Although he acknowledged that there was no substitute for "comprehensive schematic analyses," whether these be from general theory or other frames of reference, he believed that a more efficient allocation of sociological resources was represented by attention to "theories of the middle range." These he defined as theories intermediate to the minor working hypotheses evolved in abundance during the day-by-day routines of research, and the all-inclusive speculations comprising a massive conceptual scheme from which it is hoped to derive a large number of empirically observed uniformities of social behavior (Merton, 1957, pp. 5–6). Such theories might, for example, emerge from hypotheses about class dynamics, the pressures arising from conflicting group interests, the workings of power and influence in communities, and so on. Merton, however, emphasized that underlying this modest search for social uniformities, there should be an enduring and pervasive concern with consolidating the special theories into a more general set of concepts and mutual consistent propositions (Merton, 1957, p. 10).

This is very much how the scientist in other areas works. Physics, which perhaps represents the most theoretical of the sciences, for example, has been concerned with unified theory in recent years, in large part because of Einstein. But in order to do this, it posited four general theories based on research data: these dealt with gravitational, electromagnetic, weak, and strong interactions. Recent research has tended to document that weak and electromagnetic interactions are part of the same theory, and perhaps the strong belongs there as well. The problem then is to find the connecting links between the electromagnetic and the gravitational theories, and make a unified field theory. Physics, however, started from the specific and built up to the general, went from the knowable and experimental to the theory. The theory was used to tie a number of different phenomena together.

Nursing, like sociology, tended to start out with unified field theory without the detailed development of theories of the middle range. Some nursing theorists have suggested that since many nursing grand theories cannot be demonstrated by empirical data, we need to extend our scope to include aesthetic, personal, and ethical ways of knowing. In part this is true. There are many ways of validating hypotheses. Philosophers who claim both aesthetics and ethics as their domain have developed logic and other means of rigorously testing what they cannot prove empirically. If nursing is to adopt the idea that their theories are aesthetic and ethical concepts, then it would seem inevitable that they also adopt the methods of those disciplines they want to incorporate.

Nursing finds itself in an advantageous situation because it incorporates so many other disciplines. It includes biological sciences, physical sciences, social sciences, and humanities. Since each of the disciplines within these fields often has something to contribute to nursing, a variety of theories are available, including middle range theories. It is thus possible to borrow theory. Nursing is, however, ripe for more work of its own on theories of the middle range or even practice theories that are similar to hypotheses at a very simple level. If we develop theories of the middle range, they can be used to generate hypotheses that can be tested and applied to a variety of situations. The more simple hypothesis like practice theory can be tested and clustered with other practice theories to build theories of the middle range. Thus the inductive process can be used to develop theory as well as the deductive process.

Actually this approach to theory building was proposed early in the current movement to develop theory in nursing. Dickoff, James, and Wiedenbach (1968a, 1968b) outlined a four-phase process for developing practice theory. They indicated the first step was to isolate and name important factors, then these factors could be related to each other, next a nursing situation could be identified, and finally situations could be produced to test the theory. Probably the most well-known followers of this approach are the sociologists Wooldridge, Leonard, and Skipper. Working with a variety of nurse co-investigators, they identified a process for developing and testing nursing practice theory which they call the clinical experimental method (CLEM). Starting with common nursing problems or concerns, they isolate the independent and dependent variables in the situation, relate them to a given nursing situation, and then manipulate the independent variables by trying a variety of clinical approaches to see what is the most effective (Wooldridge et al., 1978).

Although some methodologists would call these hypotheses, others call them theories. Many of these practice theories have related to patient teaching as an approach to lessening stress (Dumas et al., 1965; Wooldridge & Diers, 1964; Schmitt & Wooldridge, 1973; Leonard et al., 1975). Certainly this body of practice theory now constitutes a theory of the middle range.

Although not labeled as theory, nurses all over the country identify patient problems and seek solutions. While they work, they have to use the well-known four-phase nursing process: assessing, diagnosing, intervening, and evaluating their interventions. This process is also a product of the conscious effort made by the profession to become more scientific. Ordinarily nurses do not systematically test or write down the outcome of their efforts, so simply using the process is not theorizing. However, it would not take too much effort to convert it to practice theory. In some instances, record keeping of interventions and outcomes would be all that was needed. Similarly, graduate students all over the country test single hypotheses for master's theses. These hypotheses could be called practice theories, and as they cluster they could be upgraded to theories of the middle range.

Thus the efforts at theory building that were consciously launched three decades ago are paying off. We have significant bodies of grand theory and practice theory; with some clustering of the practice theory, we could develop more theories of a middle range. Probably our efforts should now move in that direction.

REFERENCES

Brown, E.L. *Nursing for the future: A report prepared for the national nursing council.* New York: Russell Sage Foundation, 1948.

Bullough, V.L. *The scientific revolution.* New York: Holt, Rinehart and Winston, 1970.

Burnett, R.D. & Bell, L.S. Projection of pediatric practice patterns, *Pediatrics*, 1978, **62**, 627–680.

Carper, B. Fundamental patterns of knowing in nursing. *Advances in Nursing Science*, 1978, **1**, 13–24.

Chinn, P. *Advances in nursing theory development.* Rockville, Md.: Aspen Systems, 1983.

Dickoff, J., James, P. & Wiedenbach, E. Theory in a practice discipline, Part I. *Nursing Research*, 1968a, **17**, 415–435.

Dickoff, J., James, P. & Wiedenbach, E. Theory in a practice discipline, Part II. *Nursing Research* 1968b, **17**, 545–554.

Dumas, R.G. & Leonard, R.C. The effect of nursing on the incidence of postoperative vomiting: A clinical experiment. *Nursing Research*, 1963, **12**, 12–15.

Dumas, R.G., Anderson, B.J. & Leonard, R.C. The importance of expressive functions in pre-operative preparation. In J.K. Skipper, Jr. & R.C. Leonard (Eds.). *Social interaction and patient care.* Philadelphia: Lippincott, 1965, pp. 26–27.

Haggert, R.J. & Janeway, C.A. Evaluation of a pediatric house officer program. *Pediatrics,* 1960, **26,** 858–861.

Harmer, B. *Text-book of the principles and practice of nursing,* New York: Macmillan, 1922.

Henderson, V. *The nature of nursing.* New York: Macmillan, 1966.

Johnson, D.E. A philosophy of nursing. *Nursing Outlook,* 1959, **7,** 198–200.

Johnson, D. The significance of nursing care. *American Journal of Nursing* **61,** 63–66.

Johnson, D. The behavioral system model for nursing. In J.P. Riehl & C. Roy (Eds.). *Conceptual models for nursing practice.* New York: Appleton-Century-Crofts, 1980, pp. 207–216.

Johnson, M.M. & Martin, H.W. A sociological analysis of the nurse role. In J.K. Skipper, Jr. & R.C. Leonard (Eds.). *Social interaction and patient care.* Philadelphia: Lippincott, 1965, pp. 29–39.

King, I.M. *Toward a theory for nursing,* New York: Wiley, 1971.

Kreuter, F.R. What is good nursing care? *Nursing Outlook,* 1957, **5,** 302–304.

Kuhn, T. The Structure of Scientific Revolutions, Chicago: University of Chicago Press, 1962.

Leonard, R.C., Wooldridge, P.J. & Skipper, J.K. Jr. The application of behavioral science to patient care as illustrated by the etiology and control of stress in clinical settings. In P.J. Verhonick (Ed.). *Nursing research, Vol. 1.* Boston: Little, Brown, 1975.

Mauksch, H.O. Nursing dilemmas in the organization of patient care. *Nursing Outlook,* 1957, **5,** 31–33.

Merton, R.K. *Social theory and social structure.* Glencoe, Ill.: The Free Press, 1957, pp. 5, 6, 9, 10.

Neuman, B. *The Neuman systems model: Application to nursing education and practice.* Norwalk, Conn.: Appleton-Century-Crofts, 1982.

Newman, M.A. The continuing revolution: A history of nursing science. In N.L. Chaska (Ed.). *The nursing profession: A time to speak.* New York: McGraw-Hill, 1983, pp. 385–393.

Nightingale, F. *Notes on nursing.* New York: D. Appleton, 1860; reissued Philadelphia: Lippincott, 1946. The original edition was first published in London in 1859.

Norris, C.M. (Ed.). *Proceedings: First nursing theory conference.* Kansas City: Kansas Medical Center, Department of Nursing, 1969.

Norris, C.M. (Ed.). *Proceedings: Second nursing theory conference.* Kansas City: Kansas Medical Center, Department of Nursing, 1970.

Norris, C.M. (Ed.). *Proceedings: Third nursing theory conference.* Kansas City: Kansas Medical Center, Department of Nursing, 1971.

Orem, D. *Nursing: Concepts of practice.* New York: McGraw-Hill, 1971.

Orlando, I.J. *The dynamic nurse-patient relationship: Function, process, and principles.* New York: Putnam, 1961.

Peplau, H. *Interpersonal relations in nursing.* New York: Putnam, 1952.

Rogers, M.E. *An introduction to the theoretical basis of nursing.* Philadelphia: Davis, 1970.

Rogers, M.E. Nursing: A science of unitary man. In J.P. Riehl, & C. Roy (Eds.). *Conceptual models for nursing practice* (2nd ed.). New York: Appleton-Century-Crofts, 1980, pp. 329–337.

Roy, C. Adaptation: A conceptual framework for nursing. *Nursing Outlook,* 1970, **18,** 42–45.

Saunders, L. The changing role of nurses. *American Journal of Nursing,* 1954, 1094–1098.

Schmitt, F. & Wooldridge, P.J. The psychological preparation of surgical patients. *Nursing Research,* 1973, **22,** 108–116.

Skipper, J.K. Jr. The role of the hospital nurse: Is it instrumental or expressive? In J.K. Skipper, Jr., & R.C. Leonard (Eds.). *Social interaction and patient care.* Philadelphia: Lippincott, 1965, pp. 40–48.

Smith, H.L. Two lines of authority: The hospitals' dilemma. In E. Gartly Jaco (Ed.). *Patients, physicians and illness.* Glencoe, Ill.: The Free Press of Glencoe, 1958, pp. 468–477.

The Nursing Development Conference Group. *Concept formalization in nursing.* Boston: Little, Brown, 1973.

Walker, L.O. & Avant, K.C. *Strategies for theory construction in nursing.* Norwalk, Conn.: Appleton-Century-Crofts, 1983, pp. 4–9.

Wooldridge, P.J. & Diers, D.K. On patients' reactions to stress (commentary). *Nursing Research,* **13,** Winter 1964, 338.

Wooldridge, P.J., Leonard, R.C. & Skipper, J.K. *Methods of clinical experimentation to improve patient care.* St. Louis: Mosby, 1978.

Section III

THE CHANGING NURSING SCENE

CHAPTER 7

Hospitals and the Changing Nursing Scene

In the past, most sick and injured people traditionally were taken care of by their families. Although some kind of healing figure has existed outside the home throughout recorded history, he or she at first was a religious or holy person rather than a secular healer. As medicine gradually emerged as an independent secular occupation in ancient Greece, the number of practitioners was limited because so few patients could afford to pay. When the first university-trained physicians appeared in the twelfth and thirteenth centuries, their clientele was limited to kings, nobles, and wealthy persons (Bullough, 1966). Taking care of the masses of people were various lower-level practitioners known as barbers, surgeons, midwives, and apothecaries. Still most people relied on the special healing knowledge of a village person who lacked formal training. Nursing was still done primarily by the family and in the home.

The major exception to this generalization was the hospital that also emerged in the medieval period to care for those who had no home or family—the traveler away from home, the orphan, the destitute, the soldier, the sick monk or nun, and even some of those who were mentally ill. These early hospitals were quite different from their modern counterparts since they served a combination of roles: hostel, hotel, and hospital, all three derived from the French word *hôtel*. A common term for these early institutions was *Hôtel de Dieu* (Hostel of God). Care in them was primarily custodial, even though such care was motivated by a love of God. This is because caretakers of the sick were regarded as earning special merit with God for their activity. Hospitals were staffed primarily by people with a religious calling, i.e., monks, nuns, or lay brothers or sisters. Most of the institutions were quite small. A few were very large and probably had apothecaries of their own as well as nurses. Some might even have had physicians in attendance.

With the Protestant movement in the sixteenth century, monasteries and convents became suspect places. In England, for example, they were abolished and the hospitals disappeared with them. The English government soon recognized, however, that there was great need for institutions to care for the sick, and the hospital emerged as a secular institution. Hospitals in England were large but not very numerous. Most people continued to be cared for in their homes.

In the eighteenth century, England underwent rapid development as a result of collective change, which we now call the Industrial Revolution. This entailed the development of machines to do tasks performed previously by men or animals, a shifting of population to places where coal or waterpower was available, a rapid growth in cities, and also the weakening of the traditional family ties. Many reformers of the eighteenth and nineteenth centuries recognized the need for an expansion of the hospital system to care for the new urban poor, but they were dissatisfied with the kind of help available to give nursing care. Most of the reformers still conceived of nursing in religious terms, so they sought to establish a Protestant counterpart to the nuns and monks who cared for the sick in Catholic countries. Sometimes nominally Protestant countries invited nuns to establish hospitals as the United States did in Washington, D.C. with St. Elizabeth's. It was on this scene that Florence Nightingale appeared in the nineteenth century to establish secular nursing.

When Nightingale established the St. Thomas School of Nursing, however, hospitals were neither plentiful nor widespread and they cared for the traditional kind of population, the poor and those without families. The rich were cared for in their homes. Medicine also had not changed much from classical times. The physician had a better knowledge of anatomy and physiology than did his Roman or medieval ancestor, but essentially the medical role was to give care and comfort rather than therapy. Physicians could often predict the prognosis of a disease but their interventions were limited, and what they did from the prospective of today often seems harmful. Finally, by 1980 the physician was able to identify the bacteria causing particular diseases and take steps to prevent this either through the use of better aseptic techniques, or isolation techniques that had also developed by then, vaccination in a few instances, or through encouraging other preventive methods such as better sewage control and water purification. Surgical intervention was also possible through development of anesthesia. Hospitals remained the refuge of the poor, the mentally ill, and those unable to be cared for by their families. The nurse training movement had improved nursing care, although it is important to emphasize that nursing in the hospital was done by students. Graduate nurses went into private duty nursing where they often worked with a physician. Like a physician, however, the private duty nurse's patients were limited to those who could pay.

Physicians and surgeons (the two often had been combined in the eighteenth century) tried various interventions, but it is not always clear to us today that their interventions were helpful. In fact many historians would argue that it was only with the discovery of sulfa drugs, penicillin, and the development of the modern technology of medicine in the 1930s and 1940s that the physician was really able to intervene effectively, at least on a statistical basis. Hospitals and nursing also changed from the turn of the century, as educational standards discussed in earlier chapters were raised. Still, as late as 1941 (beginning of World War II), the 12-hour day, six-day week was not uncommon in nursing.

As medicine grew more sophisticated, operations that had been done in the physician's office moved into the hospital, and as hospitals began to use more and more graduate nurses, it was realized that the hospital care could save lives. Encouraging this was the development of hospital insurance, such as Blue Cross in the 1930s, which reimbursed patients for procedures done in hospitals but not in the home or in a physician's office. Procedures that traditionally had taken place in the home, such as childbirth, moved in the hospital setting. Although the medical (and nursing) profession argued that the hospital gave a better backup and support system for the mother or infant in distress, that did not mean that hospitalization was always good for the patient. It did, however, allow a physician to concentrate his patients and thereby handle more. It also moved the graduate nurse into the hospital and demanded more sophisticated care than a student nurse could perform. It is important to remember, however, that many of the things that happened with the new technologies had some negative side effects. Perhaps an effective illustration of this is the whole area of childbirth.

Sixty years ago most infants were born at home, many of them delivered by midwives. There was little prenatal care and often the midwife was only called in at the last minute. Midwives, however, were already being outlawed in most states and the physician–obstetrician was moving into a position of dominance. One reason for this was that the physician–obstetrician could give anesthesia to lessen the pain, something that was much desired by women in labor. Physicians theoretically also had the technical skill and knowledge to intervene in difficult births; traditionally, even the midwives had called them in when they ran into trouble. The physicians, however, could not normally stay in the home for the long hours that the midwife had. It simply was not economically possible and so the physician often worked with a nurse. The logical next step was to bring the women to the hospital where the support services were and where the physician could delay his entrance until fairly late in the birth process. This shifted even more of the care to the nurse. However, to win over patients from the midwives it was not enough for physicians to argue that the hospital was safer, or that it was more convenient for them, or that better support service was available. They also had to emphasize the great dangers of pregnancy. In the minds of some physicians, pregnancy became a life-threatening disease in which all kinds of interventions were justified in order to lessen the dangers. Many physicians routinely induced labor when they thought it was time the mother should deliver, whether or not she had any signs of labor. Since one of the marks of a physician–obstetrician, as distinguished from the midwife, was the physician's ability to lessen the pain, many took to giving massive doses of analgesics and anesthesia. In fact, in a large number of cases (depending on the attending physician), women were given so much anesthesia and were so relaxed that they could not bear down during the delivery process. This led attending physicians to use high forceps to enter the uterus and pull the baby out. Others used different methods which put the baby at risk.

One of the most famous obstetricians of this era was Irving W. Potter of Buffalo, New York, who turned to internal podalic version as a solution and pulled out babies by their feet. He bragged that he could deliver a baby within two hours of the mother's first timed labor contraction and that she would not feel anything. To make good on his boast, Potter developed a glove that would enable him to keep a sterile field while he put his hand and arm into the uterus. Then by pulling gently on the feet and manipulating the fetus with his other hand on the outside, he would turn the baby around so he could pull it out. He delivered over 20,000 babies that way between 1915 and 1950 (Bullough & Groeger, 1982). Inevitably the babies that Potter and his contemporaries delivered under such heavy anesthesia would now be regarded as at high risk and would have scored very low on the APGAR scale. Most were born blue because the heavy anesthesia made it difficult to get them to breathe. Their cry was delayed and weak because they were so drugged. Often their limbs were broken. The forceps that others used left marks on the babies' heads. Still we looked on these as more acceptable ways of delivering than with a midwife because the hospital setting and the presence of the obstetrician allowed for greater medical intervention.

Hospitals led to other developments in delivery. Because the attending physician was often late, there was an attempt to keep the father and the family away from the mother so they would be unaware. It was also argued that the chances of infection would be greater if the father were present. Mothers were discouraged from nursing their infants, and the hospital hindered instead of encouraged such things as the maternal-infant bonding that is now regarded as important. The natural childbirth movement, which began about 30 years ago and ultimately has resulted in significant changes, was initially opposed by most of the medical community.

Increasingly we have come as close to the midwife setting in the hospital as we can without returning birth to the house. We have restored the birth process to a family setting through the presence of the father, and in institutions, other members of the family. Nurse midwives have reappeared as a real force and have been important in developing birthing centers and family rooms. Nurses, opposed to mothers nursing their infant 40 years ago, are now most supportive of it.

Obviously modern obstetrics affords many more back-up services as well as better prenatal care through development of technologies that enable us to anticipate when there might be a troublesome delivery. Generally we now educate mothers better so that they can actively participate in the birthing process, and we accept a willingness and a desire of the husband to be part of the procedure. This list could go on, as medicine has shifted from a care and comfort profession to a therapeutic one, from a prescriptive one to one in which the patient is also recognized as having rights.

Medicine has also become more specialized. The general special-ties began to appear in significant numbers about 50 years ago with such practitioners as obstetricians, pediatricians, radiologists, etc., but in the past two decades, specialization has continued to break down within the general specialties. Thus we now have pediatric surgeons, pediatric dermatologists, pediatric urologists, pediatric psychiatrists, etc. Surgery, one of the older specialties, breaks itself down by body parts, and these grow increasingly more refined. In fact, the problem is that specialties impinge upon one another and at times the patient needs a kind of special advocate among the physicians to look to the overall patient rather than the particular body system that each specialist is concerned with. As medicine has become more and more specialized, the hospital has also become more important because it is in the hospital setting that the specialists meet. The whole manner of treating illness has changed from a one-on-one relationship to a series of contacts with a variety of specialists.

Accelerating the change is the change in the hospitals. Hospitals are no longer charitable institutions but often profit-making ones. This is in part because of the widespread dissemination of health insurance but also because of increasing government support of health care. The results of this intervention have led to what Arnold S. Relman, editor of the *New England Journal of Medicine,* called the *"medical industrial complex"* (Relman, 1980). The term gives new meaning to a warning issued by former President Dwight D. Eisenhower at the end of his term of office (1953–1961) about the growth of the military industrial complex. Eisenhower was concerned because the military industrial complex had been built up by the government in collaboration with private industry largely on the cost-plus basis; that is, industry had been guaranteed a profit for all of its military work, and there was little desire or need to cut cost, consider less costly or more effective alternatives, or even analyze how much of a defense industry the United States might need. Once started, it fueled itself and the government, the military, and industry were all working together and industry was becoming rich and lazy as a result.

According to Relman, the same thing has happened in the medical field, as private industry, largely on a cost-plus basis through government-guaranteed insurance policies, has begun to gain great wealth from the health field, although there is still little examination of just how much the patient is benefiting. Relman used the term medical industrial complex to describe the most rapidly growing segment of the nation's economy: proprietary hospitals, proprietary nursing homes and clnics, and diagnostic laboratories, which in 1979 together grossed an estimated 40 billion dollars. Relman estimated that about 1,000 hospitals were run for profit, about 15% of the non-governmental acute-care facilities. Since then the percentage has increased. In 1983 there were 256 multihospital systems that owned, leased, sponsored, or contract managed two or more hospitals (AHA, 1983). Shares in the industry's five largest companies—Hospital Corporation of America, Humana, Inc., American Medical International, National Medical Enterprises, Inc., and the Lifemark Corporation—doubled in value between 1982 and 1983. The five companies owned some 430 hospitals between them and their growth rate of more than 30% a year for the past five years is expected to be nearly maintained for the next five years (Taking a look, 1983).

What is true of the hospitals is also true of other aspects of the health care system. Approximately 77% of the 10,000 nursing homes operate for profit, and one-third of the diagnostic laboratories are run by profit-making companies. National Medical Enterprises is the most diversified of the major hospital management companies and it has a large Wall Street following. It is a leading operator of nursing homes and income health service companies, in addition to the 94 intensive care and psychiatric hospitals that it operates. It averaged an income of $166,000 per bed in its hospital in 1982 and its pretax return on assets was 26%, a figure that is hard to beat in other investments.

Even those hospitals not run for profit turn many of their activities to profit-making companies to order supplies, provide services, or do other necessary tasks. Often the profit-making corporation and the nonprofit hospital are run by the same individuals, and so if profit is not made on the hospital, profit is made on the lab services, x-ray services, CAT scans, pharmacies, and other things that take place in the hospital. In 1981, for example, 40% of the patients on hemodialysis were customers of profit-making units, something that was first made possible by the 1972 amendment to the Social Security Act that provided dialysis services to anyone needing them. Anyone who still thinks that hospitals are charitable institutions should attempt to enter one without either a health insurance policy, cash in hand, good credit card, or similar guarantee of reimbursement. Many demand cash in advance. The result is that the private hospitals and even many of the nonprofit hospitals that are privately operated are "skimming the cream" off the patient populations, catering to middle-class and affluent patients with acute problems while leaving more difficult and labor-intensive cases to the government sector. Even those hospitals which remain nonprofit are not necessarily nonprofit in the traditional sense of the term. It only means that they do not declare dividends. Excess monies are used for salaries, perquisites for staff, equipment, support, and the would-be profits are drained off through contracting of services to profit-oriented partnerships or companies. Anesthesia, for example, is often contracted to a group of physicians, as is x-ray, operation of the emergency room, and in fact almost any aspect of hospital care. Even nursing service is sometimes contracted out to profit-making suppliers, theoretically on the grounds that it is cheaper to do so, but the end result is to bring about the greatest profit-making activities to the profit-making companies.

Hospital nursing has not been immune to these changes. It too has become increasingly specialized. Nursing, however, remains the key to the success of patient care because hospitals, whatever else they might claim to be, remain primarily a care-giving institution. A whole host of clinical specialties have emerged. Coronary-care units were the model for many of these new specialties and evolved during the 1960s when it was realized that most postmyocardial infarction deaths were due to cardiac arrhythmias, and that a significant number of lives could be saved if the aberrant rhythms could be converted back to normal rhythms. Staffing coronary units with full-time physicians was briefly considered because diagnosing and treating an arrhythmia is clearly a complex function, but it simply was not economically feasible. Nurses were given advanced preparation and soon staffed all the units.

The success of the specialized coronary units in cutting the death rate attributable to heart attacks encouraged other special nursing wards. Units quickly appeared devoted to patients suffering from burns, from trauma, from renal problems, from respiratory problems, all of which represented a significant incursion into what was formerly considered medical territory.

Other specialties developed as master's degree specialization grew. Clinical nurse specialists were defined by the ANA Congress for Nursing Practice in 1974 (ANA, 1974). Although there was some difficulty in establishing a special identity and role, those in psychiatric and mental health settings were able to do so much more rapidly than those in medical–surgical or maternal–child health. Other specialties that had been on the fringe of nursing, such as nurse anesthetist, moved back into the university setting and began receiving master's degrees in nursing. Support for this expanded role was given by the United States government through grants-in-aid for training and through development of program goals (Bullough & Bullough, 1977).

These rapid changes in the hospital setting have forced a rethinking of the education of nurses, of the tasks that nurses do. This is not easy to do, and in fact, wherever nursing has been undergoing change there has been harsh criticism both from within nursing and from without. For example, as nursing first began efforts to replace students in hospitals with registered nurses, their actions were denounced by the famed Charles Mayo, the founder of Mayo Clinic in Rochester, Minnesota. Even though physicians were upgrading and changing their roles, turning increasingly to hospitals, Mayo seemed to feel that nurses should remain the same. He denounced those nurses who advocated change in nursing for losing sight of the real impulse of their profession:

> . . . the alleviation of the pain of the world. Ministration to the sick and dying can not be bound by hard-and-fast laws. They are the divine right of the poor as well as the rich. A prohibitive price cannot

be put upon them. And that is what the nurses are doing. Too great a
commercialization of their services is making proper care of the sick
impossible for those in moderate circumstances. (Parkhurst, 1921)

His solution was to lower educational standards, abolish the requirement that nursing schools had for admitting only high school
graduates, and instead train subnurses to do the work of what he felt
were overeducated nurses. If nursing had followed Mayo's prescription, medicine itself would have been severely handicapped. Nursing
had to upgrade itself in order to keep up with changes. It is now in the
process of redirecting itself to meet the new changes. Inevitably there
are still denunciations.

A good example is the denunciation of the educational background of the new generation of nurses by Alice C. Ream, a retired
nurse, in 1982. Ream, whose generation of nurses was denounced by
Mayo, denounced the new generation in much the same terms. She
was especially concerned about the college-educated nurses; she was
fearful that they no longer had to spend so much of their training time
caring for patients. She held that at one time student nurses had 3,500
to 5,000 hours of patient care before receiving their diploma but now
they had only a small fraction of that, less than 10% in many cases.
Nurse educators were her villains as well as Dr. Mayo's.

Nurse educators have a bug in their ears about being handmaidens to
physicians. They are, for some unknown reason, ashamed of being
nurses. Ashamed of bathing the sick? How else does one check for
skin turgor, rashes and ulceration? Ashamed of handling excreta?
How does one arrive at firsthand knowledge of output or the
possibility of intestinal bleeding? Not willing to carry a food tray?
How does one assess the patient's appetite and potential need for
supplemental nourishment? . . . So nurses end up as cocktail
waitresses, clerks in stores or real-estate salesladies. That is called
"burnout." Translated, it means that the nurse was not trained to
cope, to organize or to perform and will, eventually, leave nursing for
something she can handle. In the meantime, we face a stunning
shortage of nurses. . . . When some of those nurses who can't
measure up in a hospital reach burnout, they return to college, get
another degree and become professors of nursing. One can only
shudder at the thought of what their students will face one day.
(Ream, 1982)

Her remarks emphasize just how much nursing remains the same
even though it changes and takes on added responsibilities.

But what do hospital nurses do? The hospital, in spite of the misleading popularization of physicians on television, is primarily a nursing care institution. This is what hospitals were historically and while new technologies such as CAT scanners, heart monitors, burn units, etc., have led to a lot of new developments, essentially there is no need to admit a patient to a hospital if nursing care is not needed. As the role and responsibilities of the nurse have changed in recent years, the substance and nature of nursing have also changed.

Although most patients are hospitalized for short terms—in fact increasingly short terms—for surgery, or for examination, there has been a rapid increase in the level of patients who are acutely ill. This is primarily due to the new technology which has managed to prolong life, although the patient population is also older. The high technology and high acuity level has increased the cost of hospitalization. One result of this rising cost has been to reduce the stay in the hospital for those patients who are not critically ill, forcing them out into the community, with the result that they need more ambulatory and outpatient care; it also tends to save beds for more acutely ill patients. Even while the number of patient days in the hospital on the whole has tended to drop over the past decade, hospital days for a special group of patients aged 65 and older has increased (*Health,* 1980). Old people come into the hospital with multiple system problems, often including decreased mental acumen, ambulation problems, loss of skin integrity, and lack of self-care skills, all of which are exacerbated by the condition leading to the hospitalization in the first place. Inevitably they require more sophisticated nursing care.

Because we can also do more for the acutely ill patient than before there has been an increased demand not only in nursing but in therapeutic services, not all of which are given by nurses: respiratory therapy, therapeutic radiology, hemodialysis, intravenous therapy; there is also increased demand on the pharmacy and on social services. The rate of increase in nursing service hours doubled between 1977 and 1980, going from 3.1% to 6.1% (Cohen & Backofer, 1980). The largest increase took place in intensive care units (17.6%) and newborn babies (16.6%), probably as a result of the increasing rate of Caesarean sections. This means we are also saving many high-risk infants who probably would not have survived otherwise.

Even the nonspecialty nurses require greater and greater sophistication. They must have a current working knowledge of laboratory values, of the action, side effects, and uses of a voluminous number of drugs, of the nutritional needs of the patients, of the various environmental factors affecting a patient, infection control, as well as the psychosocial need of the patients and their families. Nurses should be capable of differentiating abnormalities in cardiac rhythms, should have a working knowledge of chest tubes and various suction apparatus, central venous pressure lines, fluid and electrolyte balance, intake and output norms, and the interrelatedness of temperature, pulse, respiration, and blood pressure. They must be able to monitor bleeding patients, apply or change dressings, determine frequency of blood pressures, temperature, pulse, and respiration, and somehow integrate and synthesize a volume of differentiated and undifferentiated knowledge into a coordinated, safe patient care. One reason some institutions have tried to move toward integrated care by R.N.s on many wards is that the knowledge base requires that kind of expertise.

But there are also other reasons for this which raise serious problems for nursing. For example, a study of five Boston hospitals conducted during the mid-1970s classified the activities carried out by hospital workers into six categories. The first three categories were then ordered in terms of increasing difficulty, taking into account the amount of education and experience necessary. Category 1 involved things such as locating and setting up simple equipment and moving patients to other areas. Category 2 included giving routine morning care, and lifting patients on and off litters. Category 3 involved such tasks as cervical smears, using electrocardiographic equipment, and participating in a cardiac arrest team. The researchers found that a significant portion of both the medical and nursing staff spent about a quarter of their time on Category 1 tasks (77% of the nurses and approximately 50% of the physicians). The study summarized that hospital tasks "are performed by the medical personnel who happen to be available, with little regard for the training, certification or degree of competence of the individuals involved" (Goldstein & Horowitz, 1978, p. 80). Some of this might result in greater efficiency but it might be because of low salaries. Put simply, the salary differentiation between nurses and nurses' aides is so small that it is advantageous to have nurses perform all the jobs rather than only those jobs requiring special training. As a result, between 1968 and 1979 the percentage of registered nurses functioning as hospital nursing service personnel increased from 33% to 46%. The percentage of licensed practical nurses remained about 19% of the total while untrained nurses' aides declined from 51% to 35% (Aiken & Blendon, 1981).

The implication is that while nurses are expected to do more and more and become ever more sophisticated, they have not been reimbursed proportionately for this and thus have not been able to drop some of the low-skilled tasks that could be done by others. Hearings before the National Commission on Nursing consistently emphasized the under-utilization of nurses:

> On the patient care unit, professional nurses spend an inordinate amount of time stamping charge slips for Central Supply, reordering medications for pharmacy, explaining TV charges to patients for the Business Office, collecting body fluid specimens for the laboratory, arranging employee vacation schedules for personnel, and settling conflicting department schedules as they occur. (*National Commission on Nursing,* 1981, p. 28)

Although many of these tasks sound like the complaint of any administrator, there is more to it than that. Everett C. Hughes in his study of occupations summarized the problem effectively when he said, "The nurse's place in the division of labor is essentially that of doing in a responsible way whatever necessary things are in danger of not being done at all" (Hughes, 1958, p. 74).

Nurses, however, feel ambiguous about the changes taking place. They are caught in a dilemma between wanting to fill all the gaps and being dissatisfied with the demands put on them. A good example of this ambiguity is the development of what is called primary nursing. This system focuses on the individual nurse who is assigned 24-hour responsibility for planning, evaluating, and carrying out a good part of the nursing care of specific patients. In this way, one nurse rather than nurses collectively or the nursing team assume responsibility. It was initiated by Marie Manthey over a decade ago and spread rather rapidly into many different settings. Patients are pleased because it cuts down the fragmentation of care and many nurses feel that it provides them with the satisfaction from direct patient care they had missed under team nursing or other forms of staff assignment. Other nurses feel it is a misuse of their expertise and puts demands on them for which they are not paid or recognized. For some settings it is obviously quite effective and given current lack of significant salary differentials, it is not expensive. However, it would cost more than it does if registered nurses and practical nurses were paid appropriate differentials for their knowledge and expertise.

Obviously the role of the hospital nurse has changed radically requiring more and more education. This greater sophistication and ability, however, has not been matched by corresponding increases in salary and salary differentials between the unskilled aide and the nurse. Part of the difficulty is the nurse's self-image. Many nurses are attracted to primary care nursing because they feel they are doing real nursing, the kind that Alice Ream felt nurses were not doing in the

Newsweek article cited earlier in this section. However, with the development of high-technology patient care and the requirement for well-prepared nurses needed to staff the acute care units and to serve as clinical specialists, the stratification of hospitals will probably increase rather than decrease. This moves nursing away from the model of primary nursing. This movement will most likely occur if the salaries for registered nurses and nurse specialists increase significantly.

If this salary differential becomes significant, nursing, like medicine, will probably become even more specialized. Although we had nominal specialties such as the public health nurse or the school nurse early in this century, it is only recently that we have moved into hospital nursing specialties. Specialties will not just be an emphasis or concentration like many of us take in our senior year of nursing, but will require considerably more expertise than is currently available in the baccalaureate program. This requires a rethinking of our educational philosophy. The key, however, is financial reimbursement to the specialist.

Hospital nursing is changing as are hospitals themselves. The entrance of federal government into the hospital, through various forms of government subsidies, the new technologies, the more acute nature of patient illness, has brought about changes. The physician's power in the hospital is gradually weakening. Nurses have not yet been able to crack the higher administrative echelons of most hospitals, but hospitals now have to face the choice of either giving nurses greater say in hospital management or dealing with them through collective bargaining units. Either way, the role of nursing will change. Nurses have to come to terms with the changing nature of nursing and realize that the hospital setting will require greater and greater specialization, even if such specialization is contrary to the reasons that many of us chose nursing.

REFERENCES

Aiken, L.H., Blendon, R.J. & Rogers, P.E. The shortage of hospital nurses: A new perspective. *American Journal of Nursing* 1981, pp. 1612–1618.

American Hospital Association. *Directory of Multihospital Systems.* Chicago: AHA, 1983.

American Nurses' Association. Congress for Nursing Practice, "Definition: Nurse practitioner, nurse clinician, and clinical nurse specialist." Kansas City, Mo., ANA 1974.

Bullough, B. & Bullough, V.L. *Expanding horizons for nurses.* New York: Springer, 1977, pp. 12–23.

Bullough, B. *The law and the expanding nursing role.* New York: Appleton-Century-Crofts, 1980, p. 164.

Bullough, V. *The development of medicine as a profession.* Basle, Switzerland: Karger; New York: Neale Watson, Science History, 1966.

Bullough, V.L. & Bullough, B. *The care of the sick: The emergence of modern medicine.* New York: Prodist, 1978.

Bullough, V.L. & Groeger, S. Irving W. Potter and internal podalic version. *Social Problems,* 1982, **30**, 109–117.

Cohen, C. & Backofer, H.J. A summary of trends in hospital employment. *Hospitals,* 1980, **54,** 18–65.

Goldstein, H. & Horowitz, M. *Utilization of health personnel: A five hospital study.* Germantown, Md.: Aspen Systems Corp., 1978.

Health, United States. Hyattsville, Md.: U.S. Department of Health, Education and Welfare, 1980, pp. 180–181.

Hughes, E.C. *Men and their work.* Glencoe, Ill.: Free Press, 1958.

National Commission on Nursing, Summary of the Public Hearings. Chicago: AHA, 1981.

Parkhurst, G. Wanted—100,000 girls for sub nurses. *The Pictorial Review,* October 1921.

Ream, A.C. Our undertrained nurses. *Newsweek,* October 25, 1982, p. 17.

Relman, A.L. Editorial. *New England Journal of Medicine,* 1980, p. 23.

Taking a look at health care. *New York Times,* April 14, 1983, D8.

CHAPTER 8

Growing Problems in Nursing Ethics

Ethical concerns in health care have an ancient and honorable history. For centuries the so-called Hippocratic Oath was regarded as the exemplar of medical ethics. Although the oath was not written by Hippocrates (fifth century B.C.) but instead is derived from the teachings of the Pythagoreans, a religious-philosophical sect, its intent was to eliminate some of the medical abuses of the time. The oath, like most early writing on the subject, is primarily concerned with the conduct of the medical practitioner, not the rights of the patient. For example, a medical practitioner who visits people's houses was to come for the benefit of the sick,

> . . . remaining free of all intentional injustice, of all mischief and in particularly of sexual relations with both female and male persons, be they free or slaves. (Edelstein, 1943)

Similar and more detailed aspects of medical deontology form parts of the other treatises in the so-called Hippocratic *corpus,* writings collected together under the name of Hippocrates. Included are writings *On the Physician, On Honorable Conduct* (Decorum), *On the Law, On Art, On Ancient Medicine* (Jones & Withington, 1967). Later, both medieval (Bullough, 1966) and more modern writers examined ethical issues in the light of the physician's responsibilities. When Nightingale nursing developed in the nineteenth century, nurses continued in this tradition and probationers in America repeated the so-called "Nightingale Oath."

This emphasis on the practitioner appears in the code adopted by the American Nurses' Association (ANA) in 1976, although attention is also given to the client or patient.

AMERICAN NURSES' ASSOCIATION CODE FOR NURSES (1976)

The Code for Nurses is based on belief about the nature of individuals, nursing, health, and society. Recipients and providers of nursing services are viewed as individuals and groups who possess basic rights and responsibilities, and whose values and circumstances command respect at all times. Nursing encompasses the promotion and restoration of health, the prevention of illness, and the alleviation of suffering. The statements of the Code and their interpretation provide guidance for conduct and relationships in carrying out nursing responsibilities consistent with the ethical obligations of the profession and quality in nursing care.

1. The nurse provides services with respect for human dignity and the uniqueness of the client unrestricted by considerations of social or economic status, personal attributes, or the nature of health problems.
2. The nurse safeguards the client's right to privacy by judiciously protecting information of a confidential nature.
3. The nurse acts to safeguard the client and the public when health care and safety are affected by the incompetent, unethical, or illegal practice of any person.
4. The nurse assumes responsibility and accountability for individual nursing judgments and actions.
5. The nurse maintains competence in nursing.
6. The nurse exercises informed judgment and uses individual competence and qualifications as criteria in seeking consultation, accepting responsibilities, and delegating nursing activities to others.
7. The nurse participates in activities that contribute to the ongoing development of the profession's body of knowledge.
8. The nurse participates in the profession's efforts to implement and improve standards of nursing.
9. The nurse participates in the profession's efforts to establish and maintain conditions of employment conducive to high quality nursing care.
10. The nurse participates in the profession's efforts to protect the public from misinformation and misrepresentation and to maintain the integrity of nursing.

11. The nurse collaborates with members of the health profession and other citizens in promoting community and national efforts to meet the health needs of the public. (ANA, 1976)

Such codes of ethics are for the most part noncontroversial and straight forward. Almost all nurses would agree that they should safeguard the client's right to privacy, maintain their own competence, work to achieve high standards of care, collaborate effectively with other health care workers, attempt to expand the body of knowledge of the profession, maintain employment conditions that are conducive to good care, inform the public about hazards, and work with others for the good of society. The difficulty that nurses have is that the ethical code does not deal with the more troublesome issues.

A combination of factors seems to be responsible for this and all of them are interrelated. Quite simply, the modern health care professional can do much more for the patient than earlier generations could. We can keep people alive after they are brain dead, we can transplant organs, we can do arterial bypasses, and consequently we have to face basic ethical issues that our predecessors could not have thought possible. Nursing has changed in other ways. The health care team is no longer the doctor, nurse, and patient, with the physician making all the decisions. Instead, a number of different individuals are involved, each with different background and training, and with different assumptions. What was once taken for granted has to be spelled out, and the physician can no longer assume that the decision made will be supported by others. Instead, the decision has to be a team one. Also making for change has been the entry of government into the health care delivery system. Governmental monies have enabled the health care team to be concerned with the patient, free to ignore the cost, but in the process it has sometimes resulted in losing sight of the patient's wishes about how drastic intervention should be. Moreover, governmental intervention is by its nature political and so political realities also affect ethical issues.

Where tax money is used, there also has to be a question of cost, and increasingly decisions have to be made about whether intervention should be carried out regardless of the cost, or whether some scale of cost effectiveness should be used. Since the patient is also a taxpayer and is ultimately paying, should the patient not also be consulted? The result has been the growth of a patient's rights movement, demanding greater patient input into decisions that concern them.

Government entry into the health care system has forced hospitals to do better record keeping, establish tissue committees, open hospital records, and do regular autopsies if they had not been done before. Once such records are available, however, it is possible to subpoena them, and since we have not yet arrived at a point of agreement on many major health issues, more cases are ending up in court. What kind of charting should be done? Since roughly 10% of the cases autopsied are badly misdiagnosed, closer observation of the effects of treatment might have helped modify the treatment. How closely should the nurse monitor the physician and other members of the health care team? Although there is general agreement that patients have a right to die with dignity, we have no agreement on just what dying with dignity means. Courts have often intervened to give guidelines, but this raises problems in another way.

A good example of some of the complexities is the case of Karen Quinlan who at age 22 lapsed into a coma from unknown causes. Although suffering irreversible brain damage, Quinlan did not die because she was put on a respirator. After several months of watching his daughter remain technically alive but in a vegetative coma, her father petitioned the New Jersey Superior Court to appoint him as her guardian with the ultimate intention of withdrawing her from the respirator, an action that all parties thought would result in her death. A lower court denied this petition, but it was eventually granted by the New Jersey Supreme Court, which ruled that the right to privacy included the right to decline medical treatment. Given her incompetence, the court agreed that the right to speak for her could be given to her guardian (*In re Quinlan,* 1975; 1976). When the respirator was turned off, however, Quinlan did not die, and as of this writing she is still alive.

Quinlan continued to live, however, because she was being fed through a nasogastric tube. Is this not artificial intervention? This issue has not yet arisen in the Quinlan case but has in another New Jersey case, that of Claire C. Conroy, a patient in the Parklane Nursing Home in Bloomfield, New Jersey. In the Conroy case the patient's nephew Thomas C. Wittemore, her only relative, petitioned the court to forego forced feeding through the nasogastric tube, since his comatose aunt, who was 84 years old, had the right to die with dignity, and in his mind feeding her through the tube was denying this. The lower court agreed, and Judge Reginald Stanton in his ruling stated:

> Most of us would agree that when a person has been permanently reduced to a very primitive intellectual level or is permanently suffering from unbearable and unrelievable pain there is not valid human purpose to be served by employing active treatment designed to prolong life. Every sick human being is entitled to loving care, but there comes a time in the loving care of some patients when

the proper decision is to let nature take its course, to allow the patient to die. . . .

If the patient's life has been impossibly and permanently burdensome . . . then we are simply not helping the patient by prolonging her life, and active treatment designed to prolong life becomes utterly pointless and probably cruel.

The nasogastric tube should be removed, even though that will almost inevitably lead to death by starvation and dehydration within a few days, and even though her death may be a painful one.

The order of Judge Stanton was never carried out because opponents of the order obtained an immediate stay. Miss Conroy died of natural causes 13 days later. Her case, however, is still in court, with one side arguing that society would never condone the denial of food and water to a dying patient, and the other side arguing that there is no basic difference between withdrawing a respirator or a feeding tube from a patient, that both are artificial devices (New Jersey reviewing right, 1983).

At other times, however, the court has gone further, as is evident in the case of Joseph Saikewicz. A profoundly retarded man, Saikewicz at the age of 67 was diagnosed as having terminal leukemia. Routine case management would have been chemotherapy. This would have led to a temporary remission of short duration, no more than 13 months according to the experts. Such treatment also would have resulted in the usual side effects and discomforts common to chemotherapy. Based on the patient's inability to understand the situation as well as his inability to give informed consent, the superintendent of the state school in which he lived petitioned the courts to be appointed his guardian with the specific intent of declining treatment. The courts granted the superintendent that right, holding that the patient's right to privacy included a right to avoid unwarranted interference in his bodily integrity, even though that interference would have given him a few extra months of life (*Superintendent of Belchertown v. Saikewicz,* 1976).

To the outside observer, it would seem that the effect of these court decisions would be to strengthen the belief that a patient in some circumstances can be allowed to die, that it is not necessary to sustain life at all costs. Unfortunately, matters are not that simple when they relate to law or ethics. This is best illustrated by the case of Philip Becker, who became the subject of a complex case involving some of the same legal and ethical issues in the previously cited cases but which are added to by his youth. Philip had been institutionalized most of his young life because of the severe mental retardation associated with Down's syndrome. Like many children with Down's syndrome, he also had a congenital heart defect for which surgery had been advised. His parents, hoevver, had refused to give permission for the surgery and even went to court to prevent the institution from performing the surgery. They believed and argued effectively in the courts that without the intervention of modern surgical techniques, nature inevitably would have taken its course, resulting in an early death for Philip. The court eventually agreed with them.

Matters did not end there, however, because another couple, unrelated to Philip had regularly visited him and had even taken him out of the hospital to bring him to Cub Scout meetings and similar activities with their own children. This couple, feeling Philip had been neglected by his parents, petitioned the court to gain custody of him in order to have the surgery. The court granted them their wish, and with these new legal guardians Philip successfully underwent cardiac surgery (Will, 1981). Undoubtedly there are slightly different issues involved in each court decision, but the effect highlights the controversy in the field.

The courts were involved in all the above cases. The government intervened even more directly in the dramatic example of "Baby Doe" from Bloomington, Indiana in 1982. The baby (name not revealed) was born not only with Down's syndrome but with a surgically correctable blockage of his digestive tract, a deficiency that did not allow the infant to be fed normally. The parents, even after being requested by the hospitals, refused to give permission to operate. This refusal so upset some of the staff physicians that they petitioned the court for permission to operate on their own. The court refused to intervene and Baby Doe died after six days. Because there was considerable publicity from the court suit, politicians of various stripes entered the arena, including President Ronald Reagan. He requested the Secretary of Health and Human Services (HHS) to make certain that in the future there be no such discrimination against handicapped infants. In response to this request, the Secretary of HHS sent notices to all hospitals on May 18, 1982, stating that Section 504 of the Rehabilitation Act of 1973 made it unlawful to deny lifesaving care to a handicapped baby.

This, in fact, was the contention of the physicians in the hospital, and if the government had stopped there, there would have been no complaints. In fact when the 1973 legislation had been enacted, there had been no protest from the health care professionals who felt it their duty to care for handicapped infants. Perhaps because there was so little response to the notice of May 18, 1982, HHS decided to go further by printing notices which they distributed to 6,400 hospitals around the country, requesting they be posted in a conspicuous place.

Although the notices stated that, "Discriminatory failure to feed and care for handicapped infants in this facility is prohibited by federal law," most upsetting to health care professionals was the fact that each notice included a toll-free number, the "handicapped infant hotline," which staff or other persons observing violations of this prohibition were supposed to telephone at any time during the day or night. Hospital administrators were also reminded by HHS that their records were to be made available to federal investigators on demand. In an effort to meet what HHS felt might be a deluge of calls, the agency had set up special teams to respond to complaints, as if "they were firemen responding to a fire." Team members were instructed to drop personal plans for vacations or leisure time activities in order to make certain that Baby Doe complaints received priority. Special arrangements were made for airline reservations. To further expedite a rapid investigation, the team members were given prior authorization for the use of government vehicles if a complaint came from the area within driving distance of Washington D.C.

This new "hotline" policy was not well received. In fact it caused a mass protest from hospitals, from staff physicians, and from other concerned groups. The American Academy of Pediatrics, the National Association of Children's Hospitals and Related Institutions, and the Children's Hospital National Medical Center went to court to prevent enforcement of the regulations, and in April 1983, Federal Judge Gerhard A. Gesell ruled the public interest had not been protected by these regulations which had been conceived in haste and inexperience. The court hearing brought out the fact that HHS had done almost no investigation of the problem before issuing the March 1983 regulations and that no hearings had been held. While HHS had investigated six neonatal centers where special-interest groups alleged that infants were being maltreated, no violations of federal regulations had been found. Instead, in their haste to issue the regulations, HHS officials had relied on sensationalized newspaper clips and a tape of a television series about death in the nursery that had appeared on a Boston television station and which even administrators in the HHS had agreed was sensationalized.

Even for the brief time the regulations were in effect, the response had been mostly quack calls. Some 400 calls had been received, only four of which were deemed serious enough to dispatch investigating squads. The only one which so far has come to public attention was the investigation involving Strong Memorial Hospital of the University of Rochester in New York. Here the complaint had not been made by a hospital staff person but an interested newspaper reader who had jumped to the wrong conclusion based on a newspaper report. Siamese twins joined at the trunk had been flown to the hospital from a smaller one in the state for treatment. In reporting the story the newspaper quoted the father as saying that the infants were so hopelessly conjoined that "no surgery was planned."

A team of investigators immediately descended on the hospital, upsetting not only hospital officials but the parents of the twins, as well as other families in the hospital. The hospital made the records available to the investigating team but the parents of the twins refused to allow the investigators access to the children, a decision which the hospital supported. Still, another unrelated couple pulled their child from the hospital for fear it was not being well cared for, a conclusion resulting from the presence of the investigators.

Although the Gesell decision threw out the Baby Doe regulations, the judge's ruling was based on procedural questions. Still to be decided is whether, if HHS follows legal procedures, the federal legislation authorizing the right of the handicapped children to receive treatment, gives the government authority to monitor individual medical treatment or establish standards for preserving a particular quality of life (Culliton, 1983). The government feels it has this right and in May 1983, HHS used the legislation to request that the Connecticut Commissioner of Health Services investigate six hospitals where it was alleged, on the basis of complaints by the American Life Lobby, that these hospitals might be practicing infanticide (U.S. asks facts, 1983).

Ultimately the right of the government to do the kind of policing associated with the hotline will be decided through the courts. The government under President Ronald Reagan, however, has insisted that it will reissue the Baby Doe regulations and as of this date it is still trying to expand its jurisdiction. It seems determined to assert that only the government has the right to say if an infant can be allowed to die. This at least is the implication of the Justice Department's unprecedented decision to enter into the case of Baby Jane Doe, an infant born on October 11, 1983. The infant had severe spina bifida and hydrocephalus. Surgeons have said that without surgery the child would likely die within two years and that with surgery she could survive into her 20s but would be severely retarded and bedridden. The parents elected not to have surgery for their child, a decision reached after consultation with a medical team and with priests. The couple, who are Catholics, reported that they made the decision because their child, even after surgery, would be paralyzed from the waist down, lack control over her bladder and rectal function, and this would further be complicated because much of the part of the brain that controls awareness was either missing or not completely formed.

Once the decision had been made, an outside lawyer and Right to Life Advocate, went to court to try to force the parents to permit surgery. The judge ruled in favor of the parents whereupon the United States Justice Department appealed the decision to a United States Court of Appeals which again upheld the parents. The government ultimately dropped its appeal, but not its plans to issue regulations. As the mother of Baby Jane Doe said, "There should be a limit to how far the Government can go" (Baby Doe's Parents, 1983).

Regardless of what the United States government eventually does, the nurse has to arrive at some kind of moral decision. How much say do we as professionals have in life-and-death-matters? Do we have a right to overrule a patient's decision not to seek heroic measures or to die with dignity? If the patient was conscious and in a sound mind when such a decision was made is one aspect of the question, but what if the decision is being made for the patient by the parents or by the children in the case of older patients? How do we advise patients and families who turns to us? What kind of rights do patients have? What limits do we put on our own belief system when it conflicts with that of the patient (as in abortion) or the guardian? What can we do if we do disagree?

Obviously we always have freedom to withdraw from a case. Many of us, however, want to do more. One Baltimore area physician became so concerned about the unwillingness of his pregnant patient to follow standard prenatal advice that he took her to court. The woman, who already had had one infant who had been at risk when born, had continued her drug habit during her second pregnancy and the physician contended in his suit that the seven-month-old fetus' growth had been retarded because of her drug abuse. If she continued, he charged, the fetus' growth and development would be further severely retarded or inhibited (Pregnant drug user, 1983). This case, which had not been decided at this writing, demonstrates the ethical dilemma in which many of the health professionals find themselves. The woman's action quite clearly threatened her unborn child, at least in the mind of her attending physician. He felt he had to do something. But does not the immediate solution he sought raise ethical issues as serious as those concerning the problem he sought to remedy?

Regardless of how this particular case was decided, the issue will come up again. What should we do? Should we put all pregnant women in a kind of custody relationship, forcing them to adhere to state standards of prenatal care? Is this not an unconstitutional imposition on the mother? What right does the fetus have? This is a question often raised by those opposed to abortion.

What appears clear is that there is often insufficient guidance to the nurse, either from existing codes of ethics or from the law. In fact instead of making decisions easier, both the law and the ethical codes have further complicated the issue and left most of the hard decisions to the individual. Some hospitals have adopted procedures that might serve as guides, but the decisions that the nurse has to make are often ones that such policies fail to answer. When nurses do make decisions about how to intervene or not intervene in patient care, they usually do so without telling anyone. *Nursing Life* in its July–August 1982 issue ran a series of questions about ethical issues. From this poll they received over 5,000 responses. One of the more interesting responses dealt with the question "Have you or anyone you know ever deliberately given an overdose of a narcotic to a dying patient with intractable pain?" Some 8% of the respondents said they had done so and would do so again. One percent said they had done so but would not do it again. Probably both those nurses who responded that they would give an overdose and those who would not, felt theirs was an ethical stance. On one hand it is ethical to stop pain, on the other hand it is ethical to preserve life.

The American Nurses' Association (ANA), worried about the implications for the public if it came to believe that 9 of every 100 nurses were administering lethal injections of narcotics to patients, publicized the fact that the survey was merely an opinion poll and not a scientific sample (How ethical are you, 1983). They pointed out that the nurses had not indicated whether they had been instructed to give the dosage by the physician or had done so on their own and that the term overdose had different meanings. The ANA also emphasized that 61% of the nurses answering indicated that they have not and would never administer such a dose. The ANA statement signed by Eunice R. Cole, President of the Association, stated that:

> Every nurses' primary professional responsibility is to protect the life of the patient. The availability of new technologies, drugs, and life support systems have created serious ethical questions for all health professionals in dealing with dying patients. (Cole, 1983)

The Cole statement points up the fact that a dilemma exists for nurses. Although some 61% of the respondents to the survey indicated they had not and would not give an overdose, another 30% said they had not yet given an overdose but that they might in the future. (How ethical are you, 1983). No guidelines can really be given in such situations. Although nurses might want to allow the patients the dignity of a natural death, many feel either legally or morally obliged to initiate heroic measures regardless of instructions, and feel even more queasy about taking more active steps such as giving a drug overdose. There is also a potential for legal liability. Although nurses and physicians are very rarely punished for any failure to use heroic measures (Russell, 1975), prosecution is always a possibility.

Whether a nurse should report or protect incompetence, or the inability of another professional to handle the necessary tasks because of drunkenness or narcotic addiction is an ethical issue of a different dimension. Most nurses believe they should report but find it difficult to police colleagues, and the nurse who does report on a fellow nurse will not be popular with colleagues. Only rarely is bad nursing care reported to the supervisor, and only in desperation does a nurse report a colleague who catnaps through most of the night shift. Most nurse and physician narcotic addicts or alcoholics go through a long process of deterioration before they are brought to the attention of the state board of nursing, evidence of the reluctance to report colleagues.

Instead some nurses try to cover for a colleague and to share this information informally with other colleagues, not reporting it through official channels. This, however, can lead to difficulties, and here as in so many other ethical issues, there are some legal precedents, although not enough to act as an effective guide to what a nurse should always do. One of the more pertinent cases is *Malone v. Longo* (1979), which resulted from a dispute over a medication order. Nurse Malone interpreted an order which read "$MgSO_4$ 1 cc" as calling for morphine instead of magnesium sulfate. Longo (an LPN) who was instructed by Malone to give the morphine refused, stating that that was not what was called for. Malone, after some discussion, ultimately agreed and the patient was given the proper medication. Although the two nurses were in disagreement about the nature of the discussion which took place, both agreed that ultimately the patient received the correct medication.

The problem arose later when Malone became aware that Longo had told another nurse about the incident. Malone then took it upon herself to warn her about discussing it with others. This warning led to an argument in which the charge nurse intervened and suggested a report be made. The end result was that a letter of admonishment was placed in Malone's official file, where it was to remain for a period ranging from six months to two years. Malone, upset at this, filed a suit against Longo for defamation, seeking $12,000 in damages, alleging that Longo had made defamatory remarks against her to colleagues, and that her written report of the incident was also defamatory. Longo requested a summary judgment before the case went to trial on the grounds that (1) the remarks were true, and (2) they were privileged because they were made in her capacity as a federal official and thus they could not be used as the basis of a lawsuit against her. Since both nurses worked at a Veterans Hospital, the court ruled that Longo's written report fell under the second claim and she could not be sued for the remarks therein. As far as the first charge was concerned, however, the court held that conversations with colleagues were not privileged, but the truth or falsity of such alleged conversations could not be determined without a full trial. As of this writing, the case had not gone to trial. It does give pause to nurses, however, since it seems to imply that gossip about a colleague is not protected but that a formal complaint sent through official channels probably would be. In effect, informal reporting might be as hard on a colleague or result in greater legal maneuvering than a more formal complaint (Greenlaw, 1980).

If nurses have been reluctant to complain officially about a fellow nurse, they have been even more cautious when it comes to physicians. The same poll on ethics in *Nursing Life* reported above found that 22% of the reporting nurses had been asked by a physician to cover up for them (How ethical are you, p. 29); 32% had been asked by fellow nurses. In the minds of nurses, however, physicians were guilty of most of the unethical practices that they saw around them and which they could not control. Some 9% of the physicians were believed by nurses regularly to make mistakes harmful to patients and then lie to cover them up. It was believed that another 49% made them sometimes and lied to cover them up, and only 42% made such mistakes rarely. Nurses, on the other hand believed most nurses (66%) only rarely made mistakes about which they lied to cover up. This covering up for physicians is frustrating and depressing to many. One nurse argued that "incident reports" were made only by nursing personnel in most hospitals, not physicians, and that nurses get the blame when things go wrong, no matter who is responsible. As one nurse wrote to *Nursing Life,*

> Nurses have shuttered this dilemma for at least a couple of generations. Until the "Doctors' Orders" are seen for what they are—medical plan of care—rather than as "orders to nurse," the ethical problems will continue for nurses.

In a sense, the problem here is complicated by the nurses' feeling of powerlessness, that they can do nothing about a physician. Obviously in the minds of nurses, physician negligence is not uncommon. Even though nurses have reason to believe a physician is incompetent, a significant percentage of them will not report this to a patient, even when the patient asks them. Thirty-three percent of the respondents in the *Nursing Life* poll indicated they would avoid answering the question. A California nurse wrote,

> The past year, our infirmary has had a new doctor who's handi-capped and way beyond the age of 65. He's had severe surgeries and illnesses, and was in Ob/Gyn when last in practice 8 years ago. He's not kept up in his field, and spends no time trying to familiarize himself with general complaints. Most of the time I sit silently listening to medical advice he gives that's wrong, and I can't contradict him.
>
> Even in his field, he doesn't take proper care, and contaminates everything. A patient for a pelvic exam is put up on the examining table, then a drawer directly below the table is opened, and it contains all the materials he uses. Debris, hair, and anything else falls into the drawer. He doesn't wash his hands, although he sometimes touches areas with the ungloved hand, and I fear that those examined may leave with something other than what they come with. (How ethical are you, 1983)

In this and similar cases the nursing code of ethics should be helpful because it emphasizes the patient. Nurses have a right to insist on good technique, to see that the patient is being well cared for. The problem is that nurses have so often covered for the physician that they find it difficult to bring him or her up to standards. When the obstetrician who was supposed to deliver the baby was not at the hospital on time and instead an intern or resident or the nurse had delivered the baby, nurses were once encouraged to state that the doctor did arrive. This is perhaps slightly dishonest, but nurses of an earlier generation were even asked to delay birth by tying the mother's legs together or other such procedures that put both the infant and the mother at risk. Recently, insurance companies and medical professionals have de-nounced "ghost" surgery, something which has long been a problem. By definition, ghost surgery has meant the performance without the patient's consent or knowledge of an operation by a surgeon other than the one retained by the patient to perform it. In such cases the original surgeon would absent him- or herself to operate elsewhere, or for other reasons could not be involved. Not quite ghost surgery, but common practice, is where a resident is allowed to perform the operation under the surgeon's supervision without informing the patient. The problem in this instance is compounded because in spite of the various statements by professional groups about ghost surgery, the vast majority of surgeons rely on others, residents, interns, nurses, to carry out the routine tasks involved in the mechanics of surgery and do so without getting the patient's approval beforehand. When this happens consistently, should the nurse report it or not? Certainly informing could be hazardous since the nurse might well be fired. Should the nurse only act when something serious has gone wrong?

Probably the most a nurse can hope for is written procedures about what a patient's right should be and what is the responsibility of the nurse. Sometimes, however, the only way this can be accomplished is through collective bargaining. For units represented by bargaining agents, every nurse should work to get responsibilities spelled out and to be able to work in the most ethically desirable situation.

Sometimes the dilemma nurses find themselves in, however, is more serious. Medicine, although it is becoming more scientific, still has many aspects of an art associated with it. For example, in the recent past, individuals who were homosexuals were often put in the hospitals for treatment. Some went through shock treatment or other kinds of behavior modification for attitudes and activities that a large segment of the population is now willing to accept as a way of life. Soviet psychiatry is condemned by many Americans because of its alleged willingness to declare nonconformists as mentally ill. This sometimes still happens with various kinds of treatment in this country, and the nurses must indicate their own views on the topic, even though they might be ignored.

One of the more infamous experiments in the United States was the so-called Tuskegee Syphilis Experiment which received national publicity in 1972. From 1932 to 1972, the United States Public Health Service, working at various times with the Alabama State Department of Health, the Macon County Health Department, the Tuskegee Institute, the Veterans Hospital in Tuskegee, and private physicians in and around Macon County, deliberately withheld treatment from more than 400 black men who were suffering from syphilis. These men, uneducated sharecroppers and unskilled laborers, were duped into cooperating with a health program they thought was helping them. They were not informed that they had syphilis, but instead the "government doctors" told them they had "bad blood," a term then used by rural blacks to explain a variety of illnesses, and were treated with nothing more than aspirin and iron tonic.

After the project was terminated a special panel was established which in 1973 issued a highly critical report of the entire study. The panel judged that the experiment had not been ethically justified in 1932, that penicillin therapy should have been available, and strongly implied that treatment with arsenicals and mercury should have been administered earlier. They found that the experiment, even if it had once been scientifically justified, had not been so for at least 20 years since many of the patients had received penicillin or other drugs for other illnesses and were not untreated as had been intended. Two survivors of the Tuskegee Study, Charles Pollard and Lester Scott, went public and unfolded a 40-year saga of lies and deceit. These men had trusted the government and had been betrayed by educated men. Each, in turn, related how he had answered the Public Health Service's call for blood tests, how they had been told their blood was bad, and how they had cooperated for 40 years with the physicians who were treating them. Much of the material about the case was uncovered through the work of a historian James H. Jones, and he turned over his materials to lawyer Fred Gray, who filed a lawsuit on behalf of the Tuskegee victims. Gray alleged the men had suffered from

> . . . physical and mental disability, affliction, distress, pain, discomfort, and suffering; death; loss of earnings; racial discrimination; false and misleading information about their state of health; improper treatment or lack of treatment; lowerence of tolerance to other physical and mental illnesses; use as subject in human experimentation without informed consent; the maintenance of Plaintiff-subjects as carriers of a communicable disease that can cause harm to others, including birth defects in children born of mothers to whom the disease has been communicated and the shortening of their lives.

The case never came to trial. In December 1974 the government agreed to pay approximately $10,000,000 in out-of-court settlement to the victims (Jones, 1981). Interestingly, the coordinator of patients for the experiment was a nurse who devoted her life to seeing the patients kept their appointments.

The patients probably were left untreated so long not because the experiment gave any scientific benefit, but because they were poor and black and lacked political clout. This lack of political power is also true of any group labeled as deviant, since deviance is something created by groups to define those who do not conform. In effect it labels others as outsiders. Deviance then is not the quality of the act the person commits but rather a consequence of the application by others of rules and sanctions to a so-called offender. Nurses have to be aware of this and act according to their own ethical beliefs. The problem is that the law itself is ambiguous on many such cases because coercion of the patients from deviant groups in the past has had the sanction of the law. In fact abrogation of the rights of those deemed mentally ill has been upheld by the courts, which also denied them due process and encouraged confinement beyond the limits that the law provided for criminals who committed major crimes. While we perhaps need to exercise some coercion in the case of the developmentally disabled or the mentally ill, there is a thin line between what is necessary either for the protection of the individual from himself or herself or the protection of the rights of others, and the right of the patient to be himself or herself. Do we treat patients differently because we have been told they are mentally ill, deny them freedoms simply because of this category, or do we look upon them as individuals with the same rights as others? Probably the nurse should do the latter rather than the former.

What becomes increasingly clear is the growing complexity of the ethical situations in which we find ourselves. There is increasing legislation and government intervention, but this does not make the ethical decision any easier. In fact, if the Tuskegee situation is any example, the government itself is sometimes at fault. Ethical codes or legal decisions can serve as guidelines, but nurses inevitably have to make up their own minds. History and case law can show us the direction we have been going, but unfortunately neither can indicate what we should do. The most important thing they do emphasize is that nurses should know where they stand as individuals, and then within their own belief patterns act as ethically as possible.

REFERENCES

"Baby Doe's" Parents call U.S. action intimidating. *New York Times,* November 4, 1983, 45.

Bissell, L.C. and Jones, R.W. The alcoholic nurse. *Nursing Outlook,* **29** (February, 1981) 96–101.

Bullough, V.L. *The development of medicine as a profession.* Basle: Karger; New York: Neale Watson, Science History, 1966.

Cole, E.R. Letter and statement from Eunice Cole in response to *Nursing Life,* February 16, 1983 (unpublished press release).

Culliton, B.J. "Baby Doe" Regs thrown out by court. *Science,* **29** April 1983, 479–480.

Edelstein, L. *The Hippocratic Oath.* Baltimore: Johns Hopkins Press, 1943.

Greenlaw, J. "Report incompetent colleagues II: Will I be sued for defamation? *Nursing Law and Ethics,* May 1980.

How ethical are you. *Nursing Life,* January/February 1983, 25–55.

In re Quinlan. 137 N.J. Supp 227 revd 70 NV 10 (1975).

In re Quinlan. 355A 2d 647 (1976).

Jersey reviewing right to die case. *New York Times,* May 15, 1983, 27.

Jones, J.H. *Bad blood: The Tuskegee syphilis experiment.* New York: Collier Macmillan, 1981.

Jones, W.H.S. & Withington, E.T. (Eds.). *Hippocrates,* 4 Vols. London: William Heinemann, 1939–1948.

Malone v. Longo. 463 F. Supp. 139 (E.D.N.Y. 1979).

Pregnant drug user taken to court. *New York Times*, April 27, 1983, A 18.

Russel, G.R. *Freedom to die: Moral and legal aspects of euthanasia.* New York: Human Sciences Press, 1975.

Superintendent of Belchertown State School v. Saikewicz. Mass 370 NE 2d. 1976.

U.S. asks facts on baby death in Connecticut. *New York Times,* May 2, 1983, B 2.

Will, G.F. A trip towards death. *Newsweek,* August 31, 1981, 72.

CHAPTER 9

The Law and Nursing Practice

Laws governing nursing are derived both from statute law and from decision law, i.e., law made by courts. Court decisions not only interpret statutes but rely on both common law and the United States Constitution as sources. Common law derives its name from England where, since the twelfth century, all of the king's subjects fell under the decisions of the judges in the royal courts. It is based upon precedents, that is, the use of decisions made in the past. When the United States was first being colonized, English common law served as the basis for most legal decisions. After the Revolution, the American body of decision law started developing as a separate entity, although even today the roots remain English.

In arriving at their decisions, judges rely on precedents, that is, what has been decided before. The decision in one case will control the decision of like cases in the same court or in subordinate courts of the same jurisdiction. A lower court will not disregard a precedent by a higher court except in rare cases where the lower court concludes that the trend of other decisions by the higher court is such that it would overrule its own earlier decisions if again faced with the same legal problem. The one limitation is that no law may contravene the American Constitution, which is also subject to interpretation, and this fact allows the Supreme Court to change its opinion to match changing understandings as it did in the case overturning separate but equal education in 1954 (V.L. Bullough, 1980a).

Within statutory law there are two major divisions, criminal and civil. Criminal law deals with crimes or offenses against the state; they are designed to protect all members of society from undesirable and detrimental forms of conduct. Murder, burglary, drug dealing, assault and battery, and other such actions are classified as crimes. Certainly nurses can and sometimes do commit these crimes, even while on the job. Often nurses do not know they are committing a crime, particularly in the case of assault and battery. Assault is a threat to do bodily harm while battery is actual bodily harm. If a nurse threatened to carry out a procedure for which the patient had not given consent, it technically could be assault. If the procedure was actually carried out, it might result in the charges both of assault and battery.

Most of the time, however, nurses are more concerned with civil rather than criminal law. Civil law involves disputes between private persons, ranging from business contracts to divorce. An important concept in civil law is known as tort. The term *tort* comes from the Latin word meaning twisted, and involves a wrongful act resulting in an injury, loss, or damage for which the injured party can bring civil action. The overriding objective of the tort law is to provide a means for compensating those injured by the wrongful conduct of another. Its purpose is not so much to punish or penalize as to compensate the injured party. A nurse, for example, can be accused by a patient or the patient's heirs or family of negligence. After a formal charge is made, the case goes to court where a judge or jury renders a decision based on the evidence and awards appropriate damages. Since the assumption behind tort law is that someone is at fault, it is necessary to prove fault, although most such cases involve negligence rather than any deliberate efforts to commit a wrong. Negligence in the medical and nursing field has been labeled malpractice, and malpractice, therefore, is one area of tort law.

PROVING MALPRACTICE

In order to successfully prove malpractice, the plaintiff must demonstrate that the following four conditions were present (Viles, 1980; Hemelt & Mackert, 1978):

1. The defendant had a legal duty to the plaintiff.
2. Duty was not carried out.
3. Damage was caused by the defendant.
4. The plaintiff actually suffered damage.

The standard for measuring the legal duty of the defendant is known as the "reasonable person" test. A nurse who is being sued is expected to function at the same level as a "reasonably prudent nurse" functions. If the nurse is a midwife or a clinical specialist, extra skills would be expected. Thus each professional level is judged against peers. A reasonably prudent practical nurse is used as the standard for judging a practical nurse; a reasonably prudent registered nurse is used as the standard for a registered nurse; and a reasonably prudent nurse anesthetist is used as the standard for a nurse anesthetist. Usually expert witnesses are called upon to establish what is expected of a reasonably prudent nurse at the appropriate level. The expert witnesses are commonly prestigious members of the profession who can describe the expectations for practice. This means that the standards change over time as the expectations for performance change. Sometimes written standards of care such as the American Nurses' Association standards of care or the accreditation standards of the Joint Committee on the Accreditation of Hospitals or even hospital job descriptions are used to establish standards of care (Siedell, 1978; Holder, 1975; Creighton, 1975).

Whether or not there was an actual breach of duty must be established by the plaintiff since the defendants are assumed innocent until it is demonstrated that they failed to carry out their responsibilities. The hospital procedure manual, testimony of colleagues, or expert witnesses can be used to establish this breach of duty.

Sometimes it is difficult to sort out who actually is liable for damage. Because plaintiffs seldom know all the details of the events that caused them harm before the suit is lodged, some lawyers are now advising that all possible involved parties be named in the suit. This is one cause of the increased action against nurses.

Finally, the plaintiff must show actual harm. Errors in medication or other incidents that look negligent are not uncommon in health care settings, but if no harm follows, the incident is not a cause for legal action. A plaintiff must demonstrate that harm has been suffered in order to establish malpractice.

WHO IS LEGALLY RESPONSIBLE FOR NURSING NEGLIGENCE?

Since nurses are ordinarily employees rather than independent practitioners, the question arises as to who is legally responsible if a nurse is negligent. There is a legal doctrine called *respondeat superior* which means "Let the master respond," or that the master must answer for actions of a servant or in actual practice for an employee. This, however, is not always the case when nurses and hospitals are involved. Traditionally, for example, nonprofit hospitals could claim immunity from liability on the grounds that they were charitable institutions. It was assumed that they could not be expected to pay judgments for negligence because such payments would deplete their coffers, thereby threatening their continued existence. Not only was this a well-established principle in common law, but many states had statues spelling out charitable immunity.

A second defense used by hospitals was the doctrine of the borrowed servant. The first application of the borrowed servant concept to hospitals in the United States seems to have been the case of *Schloendorff v. Society of New York Hospital* (1914). In this case, a distinction was made between the administrative tasks of hospital nurses and their delegated medical functions. This judgment made nurses responsible to the hospital for administrative tasks as servants of the hospital but considered them servants of the physician when they carried out medical tasks (*Schloendorff v. Society of New York Hospital,* 1914; Viles, 1980). Because the physician did not pay the hospital nursing staff, the nurses technically became borrowed servants. Sometimes this doctrine is termed the "Captain of the Ship Doctrine," with the physician regarded as captain. An example of the use of this doctrine occurred in the 1950s in a case involving a nurse who, in compliance with instructions from an obstetrician, applied pressure to the chest wall of a patient in the delivery room and cracked her ribs. As captain of the ship, the obstetrician was found liable for the actions of the nurse and the hospital, and the nurse escaped liability (*Minogue v. Rutland Hospital,* 1956; Trandel-Korenchuk & Trandel-Korenchuk, 1982).

The effect of such a doctrine was to allow hospitals to conceptualize themselves as only offering hotel services for patients in order for physicians to carry out their work of healing. Obviously such an idea of hospitals had little correlation with reality. As the insurance industry grew, this situation changed in part because charitable institutions could protect themselves by buying insurance. In addition, all kinds of charitable nonprofit groups tried to take advantage of the lack of legal liability. Consequently, legislatures repealed or altered state laws to allow limited liability for charitable institutions, and in 1945 the Federal Tort Claims Act was enacted, allowing suits for negligence against such institutions (Creighton, 1980).

Courts do not operate in a vacuum, and as public perceptions changed, so did those of the court. The landmark case was the one of *Bing v. Thunig,* which held a hospital responsible for burns sustained by a patient as a result of a surgical prep performed by two hospital nurses (*Bing v. Thunig,* 1957). In its ruling on this case, the court explained that present day hospitals did more than furnish facilities for treatment; they also furnished treatment, a judgment that conformed more to the reality of what hospitals did than earlier ones.

In 1965 the Darling case went even further in establishing hospitals as liable for patient care. The plaintiff, who fractured his leg playing football, was taken to a local hospital where he was treated by a general practitioner with traction and a plaster cast. The cast was applied without stockinette or padding. It was also evidently too tight since the patient's toes became swollen, painful, and dark. When this was called to the physician's attention, he ignored it for a time but eventually notched and split the cast. After this was done, blood and foul-smelling drainage were noted by the nursing staff. Eventually the patient was taken to another hospital where his leg was amputated. The hospital offered the traditional defenses, arguing it was a charitable institution and the doctor was responsible for all care, but these arguments were rejected by the court. Written standards of care, including those from the JCAH accreditation process and state licensure were used to establish the duty of the hospital, and the hospital was cited for failing to meet these standards.

The case established a new duty for nurses, that of informing the hospital administration of any deviation from the norms of good physician care. The court held the hospital and its nurses negligent because there were not enough trained nurses capable of recognizing the gangrenous condition of the leg; the nurses did not test the circulation in the patient's foot frequently enough; they did not realize the developing symptoms were dangerous; they did not call hospital authorities when the attending physician failed to act (*Darling v. Charleston Community Hospital,* 1965; The Darling case, 1968; The Darling case revisited, 1968; Murchison & Nichols, 1970).

A more recent West Virginia case reiterated these findings. In this case, the patient entered the hospital with a fractured wrist. During his hospital stay, an infection developed; his arm became swollen, turned black, and had a foul-smelling drainage. He became feverish, unable to retain oral antibiotics, and finally delirious. While he survived, his arm had to be amputated. The nursing staff reported these symptoms to the treating physician, but he failed to act. The jury found, and the appellate court upheld the fact, that the hospital was negligent because the nurses did not report the failure of the attending physician to his department chairman. The nursing procedure manual called for this further reporting, so simply accepting the patient's deteriorating condition was considered negligent (*Utter v. United Hospital Center, Inc.,* 1977).

These cases expand the responsibilities of hospital staffs to include not only accountability for their own actions but also an added expectation that they will serve as patient advocates. This represents a radical change from past practices when physicians often carried the responsibility for their own actions plus those of nurses and other members of hospital staffs.

THE MALPRACTICE CRISIS

In spite of this trend, physicians still carry a heavier burden for malpractice claims than hospitals or nurses. A survey of the closed-claims cases from 1975 to 1978 by Curran (1981) found that although the majority of the claims were made by hospitalized patients, the attending physicians were still the primary defendants. Physicians paid indemnity in 71% of the claims, hospitals paid in 25% of the cases, while nurses or other health professionals paid in only 4% of the cases. Curran also found that in spite of the decisions against physicians in a few cases, juries continue to favor physician and hospital defendants in at least 80% of the cases. He argued that lay juries are not overly sympathetic with plaintiffs. In short, plaintiffs really had to prove malpractice to win judgments (Curran, 1981).

A study done by Campazzi (1980) focused on cases involving nurses. She examined all of the cases that had reached an appeal court during the decade from 1967 to 1977. Of the total 1,696 cases involving the health field, only 390 of the cases mentioned a nurse, nursing care, or nursing service. The majority (88%) of the cases occurred in hospitals, 5% took place in nursing homes, 4% in psychiatric hospitals, and 3% in doctors' offices.

When she tabulated the defendants, she noted 390 first-named defendants and 295 codefendants making a total of 685 defendants in 390 cases. Hospitals were defendants in 75% of the cases, physicians in 53% of the cases, insurance carriers in 11% of the cases, and nurses in 12% of the cases. Approximately half of the cases involving nurses were lost. In seven cases, there were judgments against a nurse ranging from $400 to $100,000.

In summarizing her findings, Campazzi noted a growing trend to name nurses in suits, although ordinarily hospitals or physicians were found liable for nursing negligence rather than nurses themselves. Problems in communication seemed to emerge as the basis for many suits that named nurses, with either patients and nurses not understanding each other, or physicians and nurses failing to communicate. This was particularly true in emergency room cases when nurses would telephone physicians to report findings and physicians would give telephone orders. These situations not only led to litigation, they also resulted in fights in the courts between nurses and physicians about who said what. Surgical patients were often involved in suits because of infections, postoperative injuries, and foreign bodies left in operative wounds. Nurse anesthetists had a higher probability of suits than other nurses. Campazzi speculated that other specialists in the future may become the focus of suits like the anesthetists, although no case involving a nurse practitioner had reached the appellate level during the study period (Campazzi, 1980).

Since Campazzi's study, two cases involving nurse practitioners have reached the appellate level (Regan, 1980; Cushing, 1982). Considering the fact that the specialty has existed since 1965, this is not a large number. It is interesting to note that nurse midwives and nurse practitioners are seldom sued, but that nurse anesthetists are often sued. It seems that the nursing specialties follow the same pattern as physicians. Medical primary care providers including general practitioners, internists and pediatricians are sued less often than surgeons and anesthetists. Certainly risk to the patient is a factor here, but probably communication patterns are the crucial variable. Patients do not see the work of the anesthetist or the surgeon, yet they see what the nurse practitioner or family doctor is doing, and their observations are often enhanced by less social distance. Better communication patterns lessen malpractice suits.

AVOIDING LIABILITY

What should nurses do to protect themselves and their employers from liability? The obvious major point to be made is that they should avoid negligence. The data show that juries are very prudent in their decisions; this is strong evidence that the major cause of negative outcomes of suits is negligence. This means that nurses must exercise caution in the care they give, checking medication labels carefully, calling for help when lifting heavy patients, and double-checking sponge counts. They should avoid working in an overtired condition or under the influence of drugs or alcohol.

A second point to be made is that nurses should take steps to keep their knowledge base up to date. They are judged on current standards of care, not the standard of care when they graduated, so coursework and reading are required to avoid negligence caused by ignorance.

A third observation is that careful charting or a system of incidence reports is clearly needed in situations where there is danger of a suit, including incidents when verbal orders are used, when there is conflict between the patient and nurse, or a misunderstanding between other health professionals and the nurse. The lag time in law cases means that most participants in the events surrounding the case will have forgotten the details of what happened. An accurate written record is crucial.

Finally, nurses need to be more assertive when they see poor care being given. They should complain about dangerous understaffing, or staffing with people who are poorly prepared. The precedent of the Darling case suggests that nurses should make sure that good care is given, even if it involves conflict with a physician. Prudent hospital administrators will learn to appreciate this type of assertiveness in behalf of patients because it will save them money in malpractice suits and insurance premiums.

This raises one last question: Should nurses buy malpractice insurance? The answer is an equivocal one. Certainly nurse anesthetists should; perhaps other specialists should too. Most other nurses started purchasing malpractice insurance several years too soon. The probability of a nurse being found liable is still small considering the large number of working nurses. A nurse is much more likely to be sued for something involving an automobile than work. However, there is a small and growing danger of a judgment, and malpractice insurance for nurses is inexpensive. This small cost to insure peace of mind may not be unreasonable.

NURSE PRACTICE ACTS

Nurses face one other set of responsibilities related to the law. They must, of necessity, comply with the state nurse practice acts. While the regulation of occupations is a function of the central government in most countries, the United States uses a federation model, and occupational licensure is one of the responsibilities retained by the states. Nurse practice acts are the collection of laws written by state legislatures to regulate the profession. Legal precedents for occupational licensure were established by physicians. With the organization of the American Medical Association (AMA) in 1847, doctors started lobbying for such legislation. In 1873 they succeeded in getting a licensure act through the Texas State Legislature (V.L. Bullough, 1980b, pp. 14–20). In 1881, a similar statute passed in West Virginia, but it was challenged in the courts. The case reached the Supreme Court in 1888, and the court ruled that occupational licensure was a valid exercise of the political powers of the states. After that date, medical licensure spread rapidly throughout all the states (Derbyshire, 1969).

The fact that medical licensure came first has implications for other health occupations because their licenses in effect became amendments to the medical practice acts.

THE HISTORY OF THE STATE NURSE PRACTICE ACTS

The history of American nurse practice acts has been conceptualized by Bonnie Bullough as falling into three phases: (1) 1903 to 1938—the early nurse registration acts; (2) 1938—the era in which the scope of nursing function was defined; and (3) 1971 to present—the era of expanding functions for registered nurses (B. Bullough, 1976, 1980, 1982). These first phase acts are properly called registration acts rather than practice acts because none of them included a statement outlining a scope of practice. The term "registered nurse" was defined as someone of good character who had completed an acceptable nursing program and passed a board examination (B. Bullough, 1980).

The second phase in the development of nursing licensure started in 1938 when the first mandatory practice act was passed in New York. This law established two levels of nurses, registered professional and practical, and restricted nursing functions to members of these two groups (Editorial, 1939; Jacobson, 1940). This event marked the beginning of a new focus for the efforts of nurse activists whose primary goal became the achievement of mandatory licensure.

While mandatory licensure was a long-time goal of nurses, dating from the beginning of the century when abortive attempts were made to restrict the title "nurse," the goal did not seem realistic until the New York nurses broke the barrier. Their efforts, and those of nurses in several states that followed their precedent, were facilitated by the development of licensure for practical nurses, the group that had previously opposed restricting the title of nurse. Employment patterns for nurses were changing in this period from private duty to hospital nursing, and hospital administrators argued, with some justification, that all nursing functions did not require the standard three-year training period which by then was the norm. The development of the practical nurse as the basic bedside practitioner helped unite nurses in a quest for mandatory licensure.

Beside being linked with the stratification of the nursing role, mandatory licensure included another development. In order to pass a mandatory act of any kind, it was necessary to spell out the scope of function of the occupation that was being protected against encroachment. The older nursing laws merely made it illegal for an unauthorized person to use the title "registered nurse," but it was not illegal for an unauthorized person to practice nursing; a definition of the scope of practice had to be written into the law so that violations of the mandatory provisions could be identified. Eventually a scope of function statements came to be thought of as a goal in and of itself (Lesnick & Anderson, 1947).

The process of defining nursing and passing mandatory nurse practice acts was supported in 1955 by the Board of Directors of the American Nurses' Association when they adopted a model definition of nursing. Professional nursing practices were defined as follows:

> The term "practice of professional nursing" means the performance, for compensation, of any acts in the observation, care and counsel of the ill, injured or infirm or in the maintenance of health or prevention of illness of others, or in the supervision and teaching of other personnel or the administration of medications and treatments as prescribed by a licensed physician or a licensed dentist, requiring substantial specialized judgment and skill and based on knowledge and application of principles of biological, physical and social science. The foregoing shall not be deemed to include any acts of diagnosis or prescription of therapeutic or corrective measures. (ANA board approves, 1955)

This definition became the new model for nurse practice acts. By 1967, 15 states had incorporated the language of this model into their state laws, and six states had used the model with only slight modifications (Fogotson et al., 1967). An unfortunate aspect of this model act, as well as of the similar definitions of practice, was the disclaimer clearly spelling out the fact that nursing did not include any acts of diagnosis or the prescription of therapeutic measures. Before the era of mandatory licensure, nurse registration acts did not define nursing. Although a reasonable assumption might be that the nurses felt the disclaimer necessary to avoid medical opposition to the new practice acts, there is little evidence of overt pressure by medical people. In effect, organized nursing surrendered without any overt battle over boundaries. Actually, by 1955, when the model act was formulated by the ANA, nurses were a fairly well-educated group of workers, and their job descriptions demanded that they observe patients, collect data about their conditions, arrive at decisions, and act on those decisions to care for their patients. They were, in short, making diagnostic and therapeutic decisions. In effect, the scope-of-practice statements enacted in this period were outdated at the time they were written.

This fact became ever more apparent in subsequent years as the intensive care units developed and nurse practitioners appeared on the scene. These trends were noted and encouraged in a committee report to the Secretary of Health, Education and Welfare in 1971. The document called for an extended scope of function for registered nurses (United States Department of Health, Education and Welfare, 1971). In response to this report, as well as those forces which stimulated it, the state practice acts started to change. In 1971, Idaho revised its practice act by inserting the following clause after the prohibition against diagnosis and treatment:

> . . . except as may be authorized by rules and regulations jointly promulgated by the Idaho State Board of Medicine and the Idaho Board of Nursing which shall be implemented by the Idaho Board of Nursing. (Idaho Code, 1971)

Following the passage of this amendment, the combined boards met and adopted regulations that called for agencies employing nurse practitioners to draw up policies and procedures to guide the practice of nurse practitioners. Thus, the Idaho legislature and boards established two major precedents. One was to define the role of the nurse in a specialty as a separate entity responsible for a separate scope of function. The second precedent was to utilize the power of the nursing board or the combined nursing and medical boards to draw up regulations detailing the role. The use of the boards has been termed an administrative approach (Trandel-Korenchuk & Trandel-Korenchuk, 1978), and it has been used in 35 states. Usually some enabling legislation is needed to set the regulatory mechanism into operation, but boards in Tennessee (Rules and Regulations, 1981), and Hawaii (Hawaii Professional and Vocational Licensing, n.d.) were able to issue rules without new statutes. The administrative approach has run into difficulty in Nebraska and Kansas. In Nebraska, the Attorney General ruled that legislature had granted too much power to the board, so he refused to sign off on the regulations. Consequently, legislation must be drafted for each nursing specialty. In Kansas, the constitutionality of the law was challenged because it delegated too much power to the board (Bullough, 1982). More specific legislation was drafted in 1983.

In the states which conceptualize the role of the nurse in a specialty as having a separate scope of function, the basic laws vary, although there are two common patterns. One of these is to indicate that there are certain nurses who are allowed to carry out "additional acts" that are beyond the scope of function of ordinary nurses. For example, the 1975 amendment to the Alabama nurse practice act indicated that:

Additional acts requiring appropriate education and training designed to maintain access to a level of health care for the consumer may be performed under emergency or other conditions which are recognized by the nursing and medical profession as proper to be performed by a registered nurse. (Code of Alabama, 1975)

A second statutory pattern involves creating a new title or series of titles in the law. The New Hampshire nurse practice act provides an example of this approach:

I. A registered nurse who presents certifying credentials from a program acceptable to the board of nursing, as indicative of having had specialized preparation, as determined by the board, shall be identified on the license issued as an advanced registered nurse practitioner, or A.R.N.P. The nurse certified as such shall be qualified to function in collaborative relationships with physicians as well as in private practice. (New Hampshire Revised Statutes, 1975)

The educational requirements and detailed scope of function of Advanced Registered Nurse Practitioners were spelled out in regulations drawn up by the New Hampshire Board of Nursing. The specialties included nurse midwifery, child health nursing, community health nursing, psychiatric mental health nursing, family nurse practitioner, and nurse anesthetist (New Hampshire Revised Statutes, 1975). This list is somewhat more detailed than most. Usually, nurse practitioners, nurse midwives, and nurse anesthetists are specified under an umbrella term like Advanced Registered Nurse Practitioner (A.R.N.P.), or simply as three specialties.

The other major approach to the accommodation of the developing specialties is to expand the basic definition of the registered professional nurse by omitting or limiting the disclaimer against diagnosis and treatment by nurses, or by rewriting the definition of the registered nurse using broader language. New York, in 1972, was the first state to use this approach (New York Education Law, 1972); 35 states have now followed that precedent. There is, of course, significant overlap, with some states both expanding the role of all registered nurses and defining a separate group of specialty nursing roles.

A less common approach to role expansion is exemplified by the Maine practice act, which allows individual physicians to delegate the right to diagnose and treat. It indicates that professional nursing includes:

. . . diagnosis or prescription of therapeutic or corrective measures when such services are delegated by a physician to a registered

nurse who has completed the necessary additional education
programs. . . . (Maine Revised Statutes)

Even before the current phase in nursing licensure, there were state
medical practice acts that gave physicians broad powers to delegate
medical acts to other workers (Fish, 1974; Fogotson et al., 1967). As a
consequence of the development of physicians' assistants, most other
states now provide exemptions in their medical practice acts for other
workers when they act under physician supervision. This mechanism
is, in fact, a major source of legal sanction for physicians' assistants who
hold no basic license of their own. When the nurse practitioner
movement was new, this approach was discussed as a possible
mechanism for providing legal sanction, but it has not subsequently
been used much.

DISCUSSION OF THE VARIOUS MECHANISMS FOR ROLE EXPANSIONS

Facilitating Role Expansion

Since the third phase in nursing licensure is now over a decade old, it
is possible to evaluate the various approaches to providing legal
sanction for the nursing specialties. While the simple mechanism of
expanding the definition of all registered nurses seemed like a reasonable approach in 1972, it has not proved completely effective for
nurse practitioners in many states. This is, however, partly due to an
unfortunate choice of words in the 1972 New York law, which was
copied in full or in part in 19 other states (Kolz, 1979; The Assembly,
State of New York, 1981). The attempt was made to differentiate
between a nursing and a medical diagnosis using the following
language:

> Diagnosing in the context of nursing practice means that identifica-
> tion of and discrimination between physical and psychosocial signs
> and symptoms is essential to the effective execution and manage-
> ment of a nursing regime. Such diagnostic privilege is distinct from a
> medical diagnosis. (New York State Education Law)

This language suggests that the act of diagnosis is somehow
different when performed by a nurse rather than by a physician, but it
does not actually establish the difference. The phrase also focuses the
act of diagnosis on the health professional rather than the patient,
which further confuses the issue.

This language was first questioned by a member of the New Jersey Board of Medicine in 1978. He argued that the New Jersey nurse practice act, which was copied from the New York model, did not cover the nurse practitioner role. He argued that nurse practitioners were making medical diagnoses. The claim resulted in a lengthy battle between the boards of medicine and nursing. The nursing board refused to discipline the nurse practitioners, but the medical board retaliated for this refusal by threatening to revoke a physician's license if they continued to help nurse practitioners (News, 1978; Regional Review, 1978; Adler, 1979). In addition, the attorney for the New York Board of Regents (which holds the power to regulate occupations in the state) also found the language vague and ruled that it did not authorize nurse practitioners to function (The Assembly, State of New York, 1981).

States that changed the scope of function of the registered nurse without invoking the ambiguity of the term "nursing diagnosis" seem to be in a better position. One state, Colorado, added the phrase in 1974, but in 1980 removed the modifier "nursing" from its definition of diagnosis (Colorado Revised Statutes).

The Ideal Nurse Practice Act

Probably the ideal nurse practice act would include an expanded scope of function for all nurses, as well as special provisions for specialists including nurse practitioners, nurse midwives, nurse anesthetists, and clinical specialists. The differentiated scope of function for the specialists means that the nursing role is being restratified with the development of a specialty level, and that specialty level is now being certified by the states.

State Certification Movement

The certification movement, illustrated above by New Hampshire, dates from about 1975 when regulations covering nurse practitioners started appearing. Then the states began collecting existing laws and regulations for nurse midwives and anesthetists to cluster them with the practitioner provisions. In some states, new laws covering anesthetists and midwives were written. In a few states, clinical specialists were added to the list of certified nurses. Table 1 shows the current pattern of certification in the states. This certification is actually a second level of licensure for the specialists.

Since the American College of Nurse Midwives and the American Association of Nurse Anesthetists are the oldest accrediting bodies, states started by recognizing national certification by these groups as a criterion for state certification. However, more recently (since 1977), states have started recognizing certification of nurse practitioners by the American Nurses' Association (ANA), the National Board of Pediatric Nurse Practitioners and Associates (NBPNP/A), or the Nurses' Association of the American College of Obstetricians and Gynecologists (NAACOG). Twenty-one states require or recognize some sort of national certification for state certification for nurse practitioners.

In some states, this certification by a national certifying body is an alternative to graduation from a state-accredited program; in others, certification by the national body is an additional requirement for state certification. The double requirement of an accredited program and national certification is the usual pattern for nurse anesthetists and nurse midwives; it is a beginning trend for nurse practitioners and clinical specialists. Table 1 also shows another new trend. Additional education is being required by the states for specialty.

CONTROVERSY SURROUNDING CERTIFICATION

This move to certify or license the specialties is not without controversy. The American Nurses' Association has taken a position against any legislated separate identity for nurse specialists. Rather, the Association argues that nursing should use the medical model for licensure, which allows a broad scope of function for all physicians with the specialties being regulated by the professional certifying bodies. This position is spelled out in two official ANA publications: *Nursing: A Social Policy Statement* (ANA, 1980), and *The Nursing Practice Act: Suggested State Legislation* (ANA, 1981). Quoting from the latter publication:

> The nursing practice act should provide for the legal regulation of nursing without reference to a specialized area of practice. It is the function of the professional association to establish the scope and desirable qualifications required for each area of practice, and to certify individuals as competent to engage in specific areas of nursing practice. It is also the function of the professional association to upgrade practice above the minimum standards set by law. The law should not provide for identifying clinical specialists in nursing or require certification or other recognition for practice beyond the minimum qualifications established for the legal regulation of nursing. (ANA, 1981)

The ANA stance against separate legislation or regulation comes at a difficult time for nurse specialists. A national report by the Graduate Medical Education National Advisory Committee (GMENAC)

TABLE 1. STATE CERTIFICATION OF NURSING SPECIALTIES

State[a]	Nurse Practitioners		Midwives		Anesthetists		Clinical Specialists		Degree Requirements
	S/C[b]	N/C	S/C	N/C	S/C	N/C	S/C	N/C	
Alabama	X	MAND	X	MAND	X	MAND			B.S. in 1985
Alaska	X	RECOG							
Arizona	X		X	RECOG					
Arkansas	X	RECOG			X	MAND			M.S. or National Certification
California	X	RECOG	X	RECOG[c]					
Colorado	X	RECOG	X	MAND					
Delaware	X	RECOG	X	MAND	X	MAND			
Florida	X	RECOG	X	RECOG	X	RECOG	X	RECOG	M.S. or National Certification
Georgia	X	MAND	X	MAND	X	MAND			M.S. in 1990
Hawaii	X	RECOG	X	MAND	X	MAND	X	RECOG	ANA Standards
Idaho	X		X		X	MAND			B.S. in 1981
Iowa	X	MAND		MAND		MAND			
Kansas	X	RECOG[d]	X	MAND	X	MAND			
Kentucky	X	MAND	X	MAND	X	MAND			
Louisiana	X		X	MAND	X	MAND	X		M.S. for Clinical Specialists
Maine	X		X		X				
Maryland	X		X	[d]	X	[d]			
Massachusetts	X	MAND	X	MAND	X	MAND	X	MAND	

State									Notes
Michigan	X	MAND	X	MAND	X	MAND			
Mississippi	X	MAND	X	MAND	X	MAND			
Montana			X	MAND	X	MAND			
Nebraska	X		X		X	RECOG			
Nevada	X	MAND	X				X		
New Hampshire	X		X	MAND	X	MAND			
New Mexico	X		X	MAND	X	MAND			M.S. for Clinical Specialists
North Carolina	X		X		X	MAND			
North Dakota	X	MAND	X	MAND			X	MAND	M.S. for Clinical Specialists
Ohio			X	MAND	X	MAND			
Oklahoma	X	MAND	X	MAND	X	MAND			
Oregon	X		X	MAND	X	MAND			B.S. Now / M.S. in 1986
Pennsylvania	X		X	c	X	MAND			
South Carolina				MAND	X	MAND			M.S. for Clinical Specialists
South Dakota	X		X	RECOG	X				
Tennessee	X	RECOG	X	RECOG	X	MAND			
Texas	X	MAND	X	MAND	X	MAND	X		
Utah	X	RECOG	X	MAND	X	MAND	X	MAND	B.S. / M.S. for Clinical Specialists
Virginia	X	RECOG	X	MAND	X	MAND			

cont.

TABLE 1. STATE CERTIFICATION OF NURSING SPECIALTIES *(cont.)*

State[a]	Nurse Practitioners		Midwives		Anesthetists		Clinical Specialists		Degree Requirements
	S/C[b]	N/C	S/C	N/C	S/C	N/C	S/C	N/C	
Washington	X	MAND	X	MAND	X	MAND	X	MAND	
West Virginia			X	MAND	X	d			
Wisconsin			X						
District of Columbia			X						
Virgin Islands			X						

[a]The following states and territories are omitted from the table because they do not certify any advanced level of nursing practice: Connecticut, Illinois, Indiana, Minnesota, Missouri, New Jersey, New York, Rhode Island, Vermont, Wyoming, Guam, and Puerto Rico.

[b]S/C, State Certification; N/C, National Certification; MAND, national certification is mandated for state certification; RECOG, national certification is recognized as one option for demonstrating competence in the field. An educational program of given length, or a continuing education requirement is the usual other option. Where the certification column is blank, there is no requirement for or recognition of national certification.

[c]State gives its own midwifery exam.

[d]Graduate from an accredited program required, but not individual certification.

predicted an oversupply of physicians by 1990 (Report of the GMENAC, 1980). Concern about competition has grown, and it is stimulating legal challenges of the specialty roles. Nurses in the states that do not certify nursing specialties are particularly vulnerable because most of the states that revised their basic scope of function used the vague language similar to that of New York rather than the specific language of the current Colorado practice act.

Because of physician challenges, the nurse practitioners in New York worked with legislators in 1981 to introduce a bill calling for a separate scope of function for nurse practitioners. The effort was defeated by a combination of three forces, including the New York Medical Society, the ANA, and its affiliate the New York State Nurses' Association. The state and national nurses' associations based their opposition primarily on the fact that the bill identified nurse practitioners as a separate entity (B. Bullough, 1982). The ANA position against separate specialty identities was also revealed in their support of a rather vague umbrella act in Missouri in 1975. The Missouri nurses indicate that they received advice from the ANA in the construction of the following scope of function statement:

> "Professional nursing" is the performance for compensation of any act which requires substantial specialized education, judgment, and skill based on knowledge and application of principles derived from the biological, physical, social and nursing sciences, including, but not limited to:
>
> (a) responsibility for the teaching of health care and the prevention of illness to the patient and his family; or
>
> (b) assessment, nursing diagnosis, nursing care, and counsel of persons who are ill, injured, or experiencing alterations in normal health process; or
>
> (c) the administration of medications and treatments as prescribed by a person licensed in this state to prescribe such medications and treatment; or
>
> (d) the coordination and assistance in the delivery of a plan of health care with all members of the health team; or
>
> (e) the teaching and supervision of other persons in the performance of any of the foregoing. (State of Missouri, 1981)

It was the position of the American Nurses' Association and the affiliated Missouri Nurses' Association that this umbrella act covered the functions of nurse practitioners and other specialists without further specific legislation. Physicians viewed the act differently. The Board of Registration for the Healing Arts voted in 1980 to request the county attorney to prosecute two obstetrical–gynecological nurse practitioners, Suzanne Solari and Janis Burgess. The medical board alleged they were practicing medicine without a license because they were doing histories, basic physical examinations, pelvic examinations, treating minor illnesses, and providing contraceptive services. The board also decided it would take preliminary steps to suspend or revoke the licenses of five physicians who worked at the family planning clinic with Solari and Burgess, charging them with aiding and abetting the unauthorized practice of medicine.

The two nurses and five physicians were all employed in clinics operated by the East Missouri Action Agency, a nonprofit organization that serves a major population much in need of its services. The nurse practitioners and physicians lost their case at the lower level in 1980. Then the five physicians sued the Board of Registration in the Healing Arts because of the actions against their licenses (Circuit Court, 1982). The issues in the case revolved around the question of the legitimacy of the practice of the two nurses. The County Circuit Court ruled against the physicians and indirectly against the nurse practitioners in 1982, but a 1983 decision by the Missouri Supreme Court reversed the decision. The Supreme Court took note of the legislative intent of the 1975 revision of the nurse practice act, the nationally recognized educational requirements for the title, and the fact that the nurse practitioners were using protocols to guide their practice. This decision leaves the issue of the need for specificity in the language of state nurse practice acts with arguments on both sides. The non-specific language of the New York statute is clearly not acceptable to state officials in that state, but similar language has been supported in Missouri.

DISCIPLINARY ACTIONS AGAINST NURSES FOR EXCEEDING THEIR SCOPE OF FUNCTION

It is interesting to note that the current challenges to an expanding nursing role have not come from boards of nursing. For example, the New Jersey case mentioned earlier was started by the Board of Medicine. Other recent challenges to specialty nurses have occurred when an attorney general has been asked to rule against a nurse practice act. The latest such challenge occurred in January 1983 when the outgoing South Carolina Attorney General indicated that the regulations covering the prescribing authority of nurse anesthetists and nurse practitioners were not legal. The Board of Nursing and the State Nurses' Association quickly moved to support the nurse specialists by petitioning the new Attorney General to have the judgment overruled.

There is one major exception to this generalization about boards of nursing supporting an expanded decision-making role for nurses. In 1977, the Idaho Board of Nursing took action against Jolene Tuma, a clinical instructor who supervised students in the hospital. One morning, when she and her student were caring for a patient with chronic myelogenous leukemia, the patient indicated that she had been informed the night before that her prognosis was very grave and that she would need to go through a course of chemotherapy. Her physician had also warned her about the serious side effects of the drugs, including hair loss, infections, and ulcers of the mucous membranes.

During the morning care process, the patient expressed her distress and indicated doubts about having given consent for the chemotherapy. Tuma listened to her, answered questions, and encouraged the patient to tell about past coping mechanisms, including religion and dietary regimes. Tuma supported her interest in alternatives to the chemotherapy, and the two discussed a plan of action. The patient asked her to return that evening to discuss the nontraditional alternatives with the patient's family.

Obviously Tuma had some doubts about her actions because she confided in the student that what she was doing was illegal and she did not notify the physician of her intended action. The family did, however, notify the doctor. He took no steps to stop Tuma, but told them to get her name. He discontinued the intravenous chemotherapy at 8:00 P.M. because of the patient's wishes to explore other alternatives. The conversation took place. It included a discussion of laetrile and even the possibility of the patient's signing herself out of the hospital. However, after all of these possibilities were discussed, the patient and her family decided she would go ahead with the chemotherapy. It was, therefore, restarted at 9:30 P.M., so the delay was negligible. The patient did indeed develop the severe side effects she had feared, including ulcers in her mouth, but by that time she was moribund. She died two weeks after the incident.

The hospital reported Tuma to the Board of Nursing. She was charged with unprofessional conduct on the grounds that she had interfered with the doctor–patient relationship. Her license was suspended by a hearing officer who was acting for the Idaho Board of Nursing. When the case was appealed through the judicial process, the courts reversed the decision because the Idaho State Nurse Practice Act does not spell out interfering with a physician–patient relationship as unprofessional conduct. The court also held that the hearing officer had exceeded his power (Tuma, Hearings and Briefs, 1976, 1977).

The case is a complex one. Tuma can certainly be faulted for not

communicating her plans to the physician and most readers will
question her support for laetrile, yet her actions alternatively can be
conceptualized as support of the patient's wishes rather than for the
use of laetrile. There is no clear right and wrong in this case. It is also
interesting that the courts were less willing to punish her for her
independent actions than the Board of Nursing.

OTHER DISCIPLINARY FUNCTIONS OF BOARDS

While nursing boards do not often discipline nurses for exceeding
their scope of function, licenses are suspended or revoked for other
reasons. Each state lists the grounds for disciplinary actions. In some
states, the grounds are specific to nursing, while in others they are
more general and apply to all professions. Utah lists the following
grounds for revocation, suspension, or denial of a license. If the
person:

- is guilty of fraud or deceit in procuring or attempting to
  procure a license to practice nursing;
- is guilty of immoral, unethical or unprofessional conduct;
- is unfit or incompetent by reason of negligence, habits such as
  habitual intemperance or addiction to habit-forming drugs or
  other causes;
- has negligently or willfully acted in a manner inconsistent with
  the health or safety of patients under the licensee's care;
- has been declared to be mentally incompetent;
- has had a license to practice registered nursing or licensed
  practical nursing denied, suspended or revoked in another
  jurisdiction; or
- has willfully violated any of the provisions of this act. (Utah,
  1979)

While seven criteria are listed here, and in some of the states
there are even more, the most common grounds for discipline in all of
the states is narcotic addiction or alcoholism. This is because some of
the other grounds, such as negligence in giving care, are more difficult
to objectively document. When the two are compared, narcotic abuse
is the most common grounds for revocation. This is probably because
narcotics are so readily available to nurses, yet the crime is easily
detected because it usually involves falsifying the narcotic records,
and so the states can clearly prove their cases against nurse addicts.
While addiction and alcoholism would be victimless crimes under

ordinary circumstances, in nurses they clearly impair the ability to give safe care and so have been ruled valid reasons for suspending or revoking licenses.

This emphasis means that incompetence, negligence and/or other types of substandard nursing care usually go unpunished by the state. This situation has caused consumer discontent, and that discontent is reflected in the increased number of malpractice suits. Certainly the consumer concern is more marked relative to medicine than nursing, but the trend to include nurses in malpractice suits is growing.

REFERENCES

Adler, J. You are charged with . . . , guest editorial. *Nurse Practitioner,* January/February 1979, 6–7.

American Nurses' Association Board approves a definition of nursing practice. *American Journal of Nursing,* 1955, **55**, 1474.

American Nurses' Association. *Nursing: A social policy statement.* Kansas City, Mo.: ANA, 1980.

American Nurses' Association. *The nursing practice act: suggested state legislation.* Kansas City, Mo.: ANA, 1981, p. 3.

Assembly, The, State of New York: S. Fink, J.R. Tallon, M.A. Siegel, K. Lynch, & R. Block. *Background report: New York's nurse practice act.* September 1981.

Bing v. Thunig, 143 N.E. 2d 3 (N.Y. 1957).

Bullough, B. The law and the expanding nursing role. *American Journal of Public Health,* March 1976, 249–252.

Bullough, B. (Ed.). *The law and the expanding nursing role* (2nd ed.). New York: Appleton-Century-Crofts, 1980.

Bullough, B. New legal problems in Kansas are similar to old legal problems in Nebraska. *American Nurses' Association Council of Primary Health Care Nurse Practitioners Newsletter* (No. 5), December 1982, 5.

Bullough, V.L. The law: History and basic concepts. In B. Bullough (Ed.), *The law and the expanding nursing role* (2nd ed.). New York: Appleton-Century-Crofts, 1980a.

Bullough, V.L. Licensure and the medical monopoly. In B. Bullough (Ed.), *The law and the expanding nursing role* (2nd ed.). New York: Appleton-Century-Crofts, 1980b.

Campazzi, B.C. Nurses, nursing and malpractice litigation 1967–1977. *Nursing Administration Quarterly,* Fall 1980, 1–18.

Circuit Court of the County of St. Louis, State of Missouri, 1982. *Chaiyarat Sermchief, et al. v. Mario Gonzales, M.D., et al.* November 15, 1982.

Code of Alabama. Title 46, Section 189 (33–47) 2.

Colorado Revised Statutes. Article 38, 12-38-103 (10).

Creighton, H. *Law every nurse should know* (3rd ed.). Philadelphia: Saunders, 1975, p. 19.

Creighton, H. Legal aspects of nosocomial infection. *Nursing Clinics of North America,* 1980, **15,** 789–801.

Curran, W. J. Public health and the law: Closed-claims data for malpractice actions in the United States. *American Journal of Public Health,* 1981, **71,** 1066–1067.

Darling v. Charleston Community Hospital, 200 N.E. 2d 145 (1964), 211 N.E. 2d 253 Illinois (1965).

The Darling case. *Journal of the American Medical Association,* 1968, **206,** 1665.

The Darling case revisited. *Journal of the American Medical Association,* 1968, **206,** 1875.

Derbyshire, R.C. *Medical licensure and discipline in the United States.* Baltimore: Johns Hopkins Press, 1969.

Editorial. All those who nurse for hire. *American Journal of Nursing,* March 1939, 275–277.

Fish, M.S. Nursing vis-a-vis medicine: A proposal for legislation. In American Nurses' Association, *Licensure and credentialing: Proceedings of the ANA conference for members and professional employees of state boards of nursing and ANA advisory council.* Detroit: ANA, 1974, pp. 14–22.

Fogotson, E.H., Roemer, R., Newman, R.W. & Cook, J.L. Licensure of other medical personnel. *Report of the National Advisory Commission on Health Manpower II.* Washington, D.C.: U.S. Government Printing Office, 1967, pp. 407–492.

Hawaii Professional and Vocational Licensing Division. Department of Regulatory Agencies, Title VII, Chapter IV, Nursing Section 1.2.

Hemelt, M.D. & Mackert, M.E. *Dynamics of law in nursing and health care.* Reston, Va.: Reston Publishing Company, 1978.

Holder, A.R. *Medical malpractice law.* New York: Wiley, 1975, pp. 40–43.

Idaho Code. Section 54–1413 (e), 1971 Revision.

Jacobson, M. Nursing laws and what every nurse should know about them. *American Journal of Nursing,* 1940, **40,** 1221–1226.

Kolz, C. *Private practice in nursing.* Germantown, Md.: Aspen Systems Corp., 1979, 229–236.

Law of Iowa. Chapter 147.55, 1980.

Lesnick, M.J. & Anderson, B.E. *Legal aspects of nursing.* Philadelphia: Lippincott, 1947, p. 47.

Maine Revised Statutes. Title 32, Chapter 31, Section 2102.

Minogue v. Rutland Hospital. 119 Vt. 336, 125 A 2d 796 (1956).

Murchison, I.A. & Nichols, T.S. *Legal foundations of nursing practice.* New York: Macmillan, 1970.

New Hampshire Revised Statutes Annotated. 326-B:2 V (e), 326-B:10 Rules and Regulations, 1975.

New York State Education Law. Title 8, Article 130, Section 6901; Title 8, 1971, Articles 130 and 139.

News: Nurse practitioners fight move to restrict their practice. *American Journal of Nursing*, 1978, **78** (August) 1285–1308, 1310.

Regan, W.A. Nurse practitioners and professional negligence. *The Regan Report on Nursing Law*, 1980, **21** (3) (August).

Regional Review. *Nurse Practitioner*, 1978, **3**, 6.

Report of the Graduate Medical Educational National Advisory Committee to the Secretary, Department of Health and Human Services, 1980. Advance Copy, Vol. I; GMENAC Summary Report, Vol. 6, Non Physician Health Care Providers, September 1980.

Rules and Regulations of the Tennessee Board of Nursing Concerning Licensure and Education of Registered Nurses, 1981.

Schloendorff v. Society of New York Hospital. 105 N.E. 92 (N.Y. 1914).

Siedell, G.J. III. Negligence. In A.F. Southwick (Ed.), *The law of hospital and health care administration.* Ann Arbor, Mich.: Health Administration Press, University of Michigan, 1978, pp. 114–128.

State of Missouri. *Nursing practice act,* September 28, 1981, 335.016 (8). Jefferson City, Mo.: Missouri State Board of Nursing.

Trandel-Korenchuk, D.M. & Trandel-Korenchuk, K.M. New state laws recognize advanced nursing practice. *Nursing Outlook*, November 1978, 713–719.

Trandel-Korenchuk, D.M. & Trandel-Korenchuk, K.M. Borrowed servant and captain-of-the-ship doctrines. *Nurse Practitioner*, February 1982, 33–34.

Tuma, J.L.B. v. State of Idaho Board of Nursing. Hearing August 24, 1976.

Tuma, J.L.B. v. State of Idaho Board of Nursing. Supreme Court, No. 12587, 1977.

Tuma, J.L.B. District Court Fifth Judicial District, State of Idaho, Brief, No. 28732, 1977.

Tuma, J.L.B. District Court Fifth Judicial District, State of Idaho, Brief, Reply No. 28732, 1977.

Tuma, J.L.B. District Court Fifth Judicial District, State of Idaho, Judgment, No. 28732, 1977.

Tuma, J.L.B. District Court Fifth Judicial District, State of Idaho, Brief (support of motion), No. 28732, 1977.

United States Department of Health, Education and Welfare. *Extending the scope of nursing practice: A report of the secretary's committee to study extended roles for nurses.* Washington, D.C.: U.S. Government Printing Office, November 1971.

Utah Code Annotated 1953 as Amended by Session Laws of 1979, Title 58, Chapter 31.

Utter v. United Hospital Center, Inc. 236 S.E. 2d 213 (West Virginia, 1977).

Viles, S.M. Liability for the negligence of hospital nursing personnel. *Nurse Administration Quarterly*, Fall 1980, 83–93.

CHAPTER 10

Nursing and Politics

Nursing, as this book emphasizes, is changing. In part this is because society itself is changing, but nurses have also brought about changes, and increasingly the key to such changes has been the political process. The campaign to gain the vote for women, the drive to achieve educational opportunity for women, and the demands for equal pay have all had significant indirect effects on nursing. It was legislative action that provided funds for building or remodeling of most of the major hospitals in the United States. The establishment and maintenance of public health departments resulted from governmental action. These and similar actions affected the development of nursing. More directly related to nursing were the registration acts in the states, the appropriation of federal funds for nursing education, government regulations on medical ethics, and even the establishment of nursing schools in tax-supported institutions.

Many of the issues facing nursing today inevitably will be decided in the political arena. The role of the nurse practitioners, nurse midwives, nurse anesthetists, and other specialty groups is in the process of being authenticated by legislative action. Although many nurses would prefer that the authentication and credentialing of the nurse specialists be in the hands of the profession rather than state boards of nursing, even the freedom of the nursing associations to do the credentialing is dependent on legislative permission. Whether nurses will receive third party reimbursement will be decided by the political process as will the nurses' right to prescribe or to receive third party reimbursement. Even how much say nurses will have over their own working conditions depends on the political ability of nurses in individual hospitals or in local communities. To influence effectively the political process requires organization, staff, and money. It involves a number of techniques such as lobbying and monitoring, coalition building, campaigning, disseminating information, litigation, and even public protest at the local, state, and national levels.

In the past, nursing has not been as adept at political action as medicine or many other health-oriented groups, although on some issues it has been outstanding. One reason for this is because nursing has engaged in political action in spurts and starts, becoming active on a particular issue, and then when this issue was resolved, turning inward, paying more attention to internal nursing development than to the influence of the political process upon nursing.

ORGANIZATION, STAFF, AND MONEY

Historically, the major reason the nursing organizations took on the character they did was because of the necessity of dealing with the state legislatures. The major reason for the organization of both the American Nurses' Association (ANA) and the National League for Nursing (NLN) was to give nursing a voice, and the initial major political effort of both was to bring about nursing registration. It was because nursing registration in the United States had to be conducted on the state level that the Nurses' Associated Alumnae, predecessor of the ANA, moved to set up constituent state organizations that could then lobby successfully in each state. This initial lobbying effort lasted from 1903, when North Carolina passed the first licensure act, until 1923, when the last of the continental states established registered nursing. After the initial registration acts were passed, there have been, as indicated in the preceding chapter, two other concerted efforts to change the nurse practice acts.

Few professional membership groups can continually maintain the dedication of their membership simply for the purpose of lobbying. In the case of nursing, legislative activity was just one of many tasks. Moreover, as nursing grew and changed, the agreement that the pioneer nurses had about their goals changed, and differing segments of the nursing profession had quite different goals and different legislative agendas.

Thus one major difficulty that any group of professionals face is maintaining the organizational clout necessary to influence legislation. Although enactment of nursing registration was the main political task of the ANA in its formative years, it was not the primary motive for the individual nurse to join the association. Nurses joined their state organizations primarily because they controlled the placement registry, and membership in the association was a way of getting a job. This was because hospital nursing was done primarily by students, while most graduate nurses worked both in homes and hospitals, but regardless of the workplace, graduate nurses ordinarily cared for one patient at a time and were paid by the patient rather than the institution. In almost every state, the nurses' association ran a registry of nurses on which only nurses who belonged to the ANA could be listed. While there were private registries, usually it was to the economic advantage of the nurse to belong to the Association registry. Inevitably, a significant portion of active nurses belonged to the ANA. In 1920, for example, 47% or 49,000 out of the 103,879 active nurses were members of the ANA; this gave the ANA both political clout and income.

The ANA supplemented its influence among nurses by offering insurance and retirement benefits so that even nonregistry nurses belonged. Still, the dominance of the registry nurses in the ANA meant that the organization was particularly concerned with their needs. Although new groups such as the National Organization for Public Health Nursing were founded, these other organizations tended to agree with the legislative action of the ANA and only argued for specific legislation to fit their special needs.

Nurse lobbying, for example, helped assure that it was registered nurses who went to war in World War I rather than the untrained volunteers of the Spanish–American War. It was also the political clout of the nurses that led to the establishment of the Army School of Nursing to guarantee an adequate number of registered nurses.

During the Depression, which started in 1929 and reached a height in 1933, nurses ceased to be private practitioners and increasingly became employees. The early hospital nurses retained membership in the ANA in part because many hospital directors of nursing were ANA members and they made it a criterion of employment. Organized nursing, however, was slow to respond to the changing needs of this new population of employed nurses. The first tentative step in this direction took place when the National League for Nursing Education, in cooperation with the American Hospital Association, issued the *Manual of the Essentials of Good Hospital Nursing Service*, which set some minimal standards for nursing practice in hospitals without nursing schools. It was not until World War II, however, that organized nursing turned to a consideration of collective bargaining as a way of improving nursing wages and services, and this delay ultimately cut down the percentages of nurses belonging to the professional association.

Collective bargaining for nurses started in California, in part because of the large explosion of population in that state. The rapid buildup of both military installations and the defense industry required the expansion of the existing health care establishment. Nurses were in short supply and were recruited from all over the country, but once they arrived, they did not find themselves benefiting in any material way from this shortage. Salaries were low compared with what they could earn in the defense plants. One alternative was to leave nursing, and many did, but others, determined to remain as nurses, saw labor union affiliation as a way of improving their condition. Faced with a defection of nurses to organized labor unless it acted, the California Nurses' Association (CNA) sought to become a bargaining agent in its own right. Immediately, the CNA ran into a roadblock from the ANA since the bylaws of the national nursing organization did not permit any of its constituent state organizations to act as bargaining agents (Bullough & Bullough, 1978).

This problem was finally resolved in 1944 when the ANA Board of Directors stated that although the national organization had to remain aloof from collective bargaining, the individual state associations were free to do so. A committee was also formed to study employment conditions of registered nurses with Shirley Titus, executive director of the California Nurses' Association, as its head. In 1946 the ANA adopted an economic security program, including collective bargaining for state and district nurses' associations. Although there was considerable reluctance on behalf of some to engage in collective bargaining, their reluctance was overcome by fear of a mass defection of nurses into labor unions. In order to gain a favorable vote on collective bargaining, however, two concessions were made to those worried about the change in ANA policy. First, the ANA stated that none of its members could join any other organization that could act as a bargaining agent, and second, the package was weakened by a clause that "under no circumstances would a strike or use of any similar coercive device be countenanced" (Bullough & Bullough, 1978, p. 208).

Both of these clauses ultimately undermined the success of the ANA. When the ANA had adopted its economic package, hospitals were under the provisions of the 1935 Wagner Act, which obliged them to bargain with their employees. In 1947, the Taft-Hartley Labor Management Relations Act specifically exempted nonprofit hospitals from the necessity of recognizing bargaining rights of employees. Although the Taft–Hartley Act technically did not make collective bargaining for hospital employees illegal, the ANA pledge not to strike effectively denied the nurses any means of forcing the hospital to recognize them. Labor unions, not willing to abide by the ANA pledge not to strike and concerned at first with the nonnursing employees in the hospital, were able to extend their contracts to cover nurses at the expense of the ANA, which then did not allow such nurses to be members. It was not until 1968 that the ANA abandoned its no-strike pledge.

After reaching a high of 57% of active nurses in 1940, the proportion of nurses holding ANA membership has since been on a more or less continuous decline, although total numbers are up because the total number of nurses is up. In 1979, only 16% or 181,212 nurses out of 1,119,100 active nurses belonged to the ANA (see Table 1). It was not until 1974 when the Labor Relations Act was finally amended to include employees of nonprofit health care institutions, that collective bargaining became an important function of the organization. But by that time, labor unions and others had already established a strong foothold in the health professions, and nurses often turned to unions rather than choosing the ANA affiliate as a bargaining agent. In some states, contracts called for nurses to join the state but not the national association, a fact which further weakened the national association. Since membership dues often reflected the need to hire negotiators and officials to supervise those contracts in states where local nurses' associations did engage in collective bargaining, many nurses who did not belong to the bargaining unit ceased to be members. To further complicate the issue, supervisors and directors, previously the bulwark of the ANA, left the organization because National Labor Relations Board (NLRB) rules discouraged their belonging to a bargaining agent.

Another cause for declining membership has been the reluctance of the ANA to allow certain groups of specialty nurses, such as occupational health nurses, nurse anesthetists, nurse midwives, and nurse practitioners, to maintain a separate identity. This has led to the growth of independent nursing organizations with agendas somewhat different from the ANA or NLN. The result, at times, is a conflict among nurses over what legislation should be enacted.

Whether this breaking-away process could have been prevented with better leadership is debatable. The ANA was most effectively organized to lobby at the state level, and even here its power has been curtailed. When federal monies and federal programs came to play an increasingly dominant role in nursing, neither the ANA nor the NLN was particularly well equipped to push its own case. One consequence of this was the formation in 1969 of the American Association of Colleges of Nursing, which speaks for collegiate nurse educators in Washington, D.C.

The ANA itself also attempted to be somewhat more political on

TABLE 1. ANA MEMBERSHIP

Year	Employed Nurses	ANA Members	Percentage
1920–1922	103,879	49,000	47
1930	214,292	100,000	47
1940	294,189	167,201	57
1950	374,584	175,785	47
1960	504,000	170,911	34
1970	700,000	181,115	26
1980	1,119,100	181,212	16

Sources
American Nurses' Association. Facts about nursing: A statistical summary, 1970–71 ed.
New York: The Association, 1971, pp. 9, 63. American Nurses' Association. Facts about
nursing: A statistical summary, 1980–81. New York: American Journal of Nursing Co.,
1981, pp. 6, 119.

the national scene. In January 1971, the ANA's Government Relations Department moved to Washington, D.C. and under its Director Constance Holleran aggressively attempted to represent nursing on Capital Hill. In 1972 the Nurses for Political Action was organized as a nonpartisan, nonprofit association to attain support of legislators, government officials, and the general public for nursing. In an official statement, the organizing group noted that nurses, who then numbered approximately one million persons, were rarely consulted by the government legislative bodies in Washington enacting legislation that dealt directly with issues on which they were expert. The organization listed as its first priority the achievement of substantive political influence on national policy relating to the delivery of health care, the inclusion of nurses in those groups responsible for the drafting of health care legislation, and recognition of their collaborative and independent functions as nurses in the health system. The organization soon affiliated with the ANA and subsequently changed its name to Nurses' Coalition for Action in Politics (N-CAP). The ANA itself weakened this positive step by moving its headquarters to Kansas City from New York at a time when national associations are increasingly locating in Washington, D.C. to supplement the lobbying power of their political arms. It is also possible that the ANA move in 1982 to change its organization from a national one to a federation, giving more powers to state organizations and less power (and money) to the national organization, might further weaken any political stance that the ANA might take.

Increasingly, the strategy for effective political action for nursing probably rests not with any one organization, or even a political action group such as N-CAP, but with a coalition. That coalition should function not only at the national but at the state and local levels as well. As of this time, the most likely nucleus for such a coalition would be the National Federation for Specialty Nursing Organizations. Founded in 1973 with 13 nursing organizations, the Federation now includes 27 groups; Table 2 shows the membership. Although the Federation potentially could speak for all of nursing, it is now handicapped by its organizational structure, wherein the presidency rotates to a different organization every six months. If current plans for incorporation reach fruition, and the Federation secures a permanent address and an ongoing structure, the organization has the potential of becoming a more useful tool for political action.

The ANA itself has begun to take steps to be more effective in capturing the specialties by establishing a Nursing Organization Liaison within the ANA. The danger is that some of the energy spent in strengthening a legislative program for all nursing groups might be spent in a power struggle among the various nursing groups. Regardless of the eventual decision over which organizations will represent nursing, it is essential to emphasize that some kind of united front has to be active in the legislative area if nurses are to be heard in Washington.

POLITICAL ACTION

Since most nursing issues are bipartisan, it should not be too difficult for nurses who disagree on partisan issues to agree on basic nursing ones. Republican-oriented nurses can work one side of the legislative aisle and Democratically oriented ones the other. There are any number of issues that need legislative action, either at the national or state level, including the right of nurse midwives to practice, the entry into practice legislation, equal pay to males doing jobs requiring similar skills and educational background, third party reimbursement, and for specialists such as nurse practitioners, the right to prescribe and enter into independent practice.

In each case, it is important for nurses to analyze the political situation and plan a course of action. In some cases, an individual nurse can be the catalyst, in others, an organization is needed. Regardless of the number or kind of supporters, the same kind of action has to be taken. In our various activities, we have developed and utilized a method for political action that uses a theoretical framework for social change, outlined by Kurt Lewin (1958). The model can

TABLE 2. NATIONAL FEDERATION FOR SPECIALTY
NURSING ORGANIZATIONS[a]

Member Organizations	
Organization	Date Jointed the Federation
American Association of Critical-Care Nurses (AACN) One Civic Plaza Newport Beach, CA 92660	Charter Member[b]
American Association of Nephrology Nurses and Technicians Box 56 North Woodbury Road Pitman, NJ 08071	Charter Member
American Association of Neurosurgical Nurses 625 N. Michigan Avenue, Suite 1519 Chicago, IL 60611	Charter Member
American Association of Nurse Anesthetists 216 Higgins Road Park Ridge, IL 60068	Charter Member
American Association of Occupational Health Nurses, Inc. 3500 Piedmont Road NE Atlanta, GA 30305	Charter Member
American College of Nurse-Midwives 1522 K Street, NW, Suite 1120 Washington, DC 20005	Charter Member
American Nurses' Association 2420 Pershing Road, 5th Floor Kansas City, MO 64108	Charter Member
American Public Health Association/Public Health Nursing Section 1015 15th Street, NW Washington, DC 20005	Charter Member
American Society of Nursing Service Administrators 840 N. Lake Shore Drive Chicago, IL 60611	June 1982
American Society of Opthalmic Registered Nurses, Inc. 41 N. Bellmawr Avenue Bellmawr, NJ 08031	June 1979
American Society of Plastic & Reconstructive Surgical Nurses 23341 N. Milwaukee Avenue Half Day, IL 60069	June 1980
American Urological Association Allied Nurses 21510 South Main Street Carson, CA 90745	Charter Member
Association for Practitioners in Infection Control	January 1977

Member Organizations

Organization	Date Joined the Federation
Rt. 2, 359 Milwaukee Avenue Half Day, IL 60069	
Association of Operating Room Nurses, Inc. 10170 E. Mississippi Avenue Denver, CO 80231	Charter Member
Association of Rehabilitation Nurses 2506 Gross Point Road Evanston, IL 60201	January 1976
Emergency Department Nurses Association 666 North Lake Shore Drive, Suite 1131 Chicago, IL 60611	Charter Member
International Association for Enterostomal Therapy, Inc. 505 N. Tustin Avenue, Suite 282 Santa Ana, CA 92705	June 1976
National Association of Orthopaedic Nurses (NAON) North Woodbury Road, Box 56 Pitman, NJ 08071	January 1982
National Association of Pediatric Nurse Practitioners and Associates North Woodbury Road, Box 56 Pitman, NJ 08071	June 1974
National Association of School Nurses 7706 John Hancock Lane Dayton, OH 45459	Charter Member
National Intravenous Therapy Association 87 Blanchard Road Cambridge, MA 02138[b]	Charter Member
National League for Nursing 10 Columbus Circle New York, NY 10019	January 1982
National Nurse Society on Alcoholism 870 El Camino del Mar San Francisco, CA 94121	January 1979
The Nurses Association of the American College of Obstetricians and Gynecologists 600 Maryland Avenue, SW, Suite 200 Washington, DC 20024	Charter Member
Oncology Nursing Society 701 Washington Road Pittsburgh, PA 15228	January 1977

[a]Effective February 1, 1983.
[b]Charter Member date was June 1973.

obviously be modified to suit a particular situation or group, but the techniques of the six-step process essentially remain the same:

1. Step 1 is determining exactly what kind of political change the person or group wants to make. As an example, the change might be the right of a nurse practitioner to prescribe certain basic drugs.

2. Once the decision on the nature of change is decided upon, then the next step is to decide the target for political example. Obviously the right to prescribe requires state legislative approval. If the change desired is the increase of federal funding for nursing education, Congress might become the target. Choosing the target group is important so the action can be pinpointed. Diffuse public relations campaigns sound attractive, but they are expensive and not nearly so effective.

3. Organizations, power blocks, and even important individuals should be listed in one of three different categories: Driving Forces, Neutral Forces, Restraining Forces. Obviously one of the restraining forces on nurses prescribing would be the state medical society. Nursing organizations of all kinds could be the driving forces, and a coalition of nursing groups could be formed for this particular group. Most groups of consumers, such as women's groups, would likely remain neutral. So, probably, would most other health professionals.

4. How can the restraining forces be neutralized? Physicians, for example, might become less hostile and more neutral if the number or variety of drugs to be prescribed is limited to specific categories. Most physicians themselves rely on 20 or 30 drugs in their practice, and while the specific drugs need not be named, if only because the drug industry keeps changing and new drugs appear on the market, classes of drugs could be listed and periodically updated. Physician hostility might be further lessened if the board of nursing worked in conjunction with the board of medicine to issue new lists of drugs.

5. Converting the neutral forces into driving forces is the next step. Pharmacists, for example, might be regarded as a neutral force. Pharmacists, however, are eager to extend their own scope of practice. A coalition of pharmacists and nurses might work on a particular nursing project in return for nursing support of the individual group's needs. Women's groups can be moved from neutral to driving forces if the issue can be shown to involve women's health care or better child care or other issues that women as a group are concerned with.

6. The last step is the key step, namely, the supporting and mobilizing of friends and allies. This involves effective publicity of the cause, rallying of support through parties or even demonstration, and teaching the public and the legislators what is really involved. If the restraining forces can be lessened and the driving forces increased, then the nature of the political equilibrium that had held the forces in check will change, and ultimately change will come about.

The format can also be used for political activities not involving governmental bodies. A good illustration of this is what happened when one of the authors of this book used the format as a teaching tool in a nursing issues course. To demonstrate its effectiveness, the students were encouraged to bring about a change in something of concern to them. Some of the students decided they wanted to change the image of nursing presented in a wine commercial they found offensive to nursing. The commercial pictured a happy young female physician toasting her father with Inglenook wine and saying:

> When I wanted to be a pompom girl you said, "Go all the way—be a cheerleader." Then when I said I wanted to be a nurse, you said, 'Go all the way—be a doctor.'

After some library research to find the company headquarters and its officers (Hublein Company), the students had identified the target. The nurses were obviously the driving force for change, and as far as they were concerned, everyone else was neutral, although the company itself was the restraining force as well as the target for activity. The nurses took as their major task the mobilization of other nurses, moving them from a neutral to an active stance. They began with a letter-writing campaign to the company among their small group and also wrote to the local nursing association and to the national offices of both the ANA and NLN. Both ANA and NLN officials wrote letters to the company.

The students also decided to escalate their campaign beyond letter writing and began to take steps to organize a boycott against Inglenook wines because of their put-down of nurses. The first announcement of this decision was to the school newspaper, and at this juncture fate also intervened. A local reporter for the wire service picked up the story and called the winery to check the students' complaints.

The results were immediate. A telephone call and a letter came from the director of public relations promising to change the commercial. When asked why the winery had delayed in responding to the students, he indicated that initially only five letters expressing displeasure had been received and that this number was not considered significant. Only when more than eight letters had arrived, as well as the telephone call from the wire service, did the winery decide that action was necessary. The commercial was removed from the air, and the committee was consulted about the content of the substitute one, which showed the happy young physician with no negative allusion to nursing or any other profession. Although not all class demonstrations of the political process work so well, it is important to emphasize that the political process is not impossible to influence.

There are other ways to bring change about, and that is through litigation. In the past organized nursing has rarely engaged in lawsuits on behalf of nursing. In a constitutional government such as the United States, however, enforcement of laws has to be based on the interpretation of the Constitution; laws themselves have to be interpreted, and this leaves the judges room to bring about changes that might or might not have been intended by the legislators when they enacted the law. A good example of social change brought about by the courts is the 1954 decision outlawing separate but equal schooling. In this case, the court finally accepted the findings of social scientists that it was impossible for education to be both separate and equal since the very nature of separateness caused inequality.

Even court cases that go against the plaintiffs can bring about change. A good example is the Denver case mentioned earlier in this book, where in 1978 a group of Denver nurses sued for an adjustment in their pay scale as set by the City and County of Denver. The published entry-level salaries for staff nurses in 1977 was $316 a month less than that for sign painters, and a graduate nurse I was paid less than a plumber I, tree trimmer I, tire serviceman I, oiler I, gardener–florist I, or parking meter repairman. At the top of the nursing ladder, the Director of Nursing Service—then supervising 575 employees and administering an annual budget of $3.5 million, and with 17 years of education and a master's degree—was paid less than 19 city job classifications filled entirely by men that required the same or less combined education and experience and the same or less supervisory responsibility (Barnes, 1980). Although the nurses ultimately lost their suit in federal court and on appeal to the United States Supreme Court, the principle was later upheld in lawsuits by different groups of employees, as the Supreme Court has gradually worked to eliminate the kind of blatant discrimination between men and women so obvious in the Denver case (Hershey, 1983). The recent Missouri case covered in the preceeding chapter demonstrates the most effective use of the court system by nursing organizations to date. Thirty-six organizations, including most of the major nursing organizations, submitted *amicus curiae* briefs to the Missouri Supreme Court. The court was so impressed by this support that it referred to the briefs in its decision.

Strike, job action, or public protest of one kind or another entails still another kind of political education. All can be used to educate the public, to bring nursing issues to public attention. The modern hospital runs on the backs of nurses, and no hospital or any other health care institution can function effectively if the nurses are not properly appreciated and rewarded.

We have emphasized throughout this book that nursing is in transition, that lots of things are changing. Undoubtedly, many more things have to change before nursing is recognized as the responsible profession it is. We cannot, however, rely upon a professional association to do all our work, or even a coalition of professional associations. Change comes when a nurse, or a group of nurses, decides something should change. We cannot wait for others to make the changes. When we see something wrong, we have to work out the solutions ourselves. Change might be inevitable, as the philosophers put it, but only through the political process can we help to direct the changes, whether it be in legislation, in education, or even in the official nursing organizations themselves.

REFERENCES

Barnes, C.S. Denver: A case study. In B. Bullough (Ed.), *The law and the expanding nursing role.* New York: Appleton-Century-Crofts, 1980.

Bullough, B. (Ed.). *The law and the expanding nursing role.* New York: Appleton-Century-Crofts, 1980.

Bullough, V.L. & Bullough, B. *The care of the sick.* New York: Neale Watson, Science History, 1978.

Hershey, Robert D. Women's pay fight shifts to "Comparable Worth." *New York Times,* November 1, 1983, 415.

Lewin, K. Group decision and social change. *Readings on social psychology.* New York: Holt, Rinehart and Winston, 1958.

Guide for Further Reading

Books and articles have been cited in the references throughout this work. The following books and articles have been particularly valuable, and should prove to be helpful to those wishing to read further.

BOOKS

American Academy of Nursing. *The impact of changing resources on health policy.* Kansas City, Mo.: American Nurses' Association, 1981.

American Academy of Nursing (L. H. Aiken, Ed.). *Health policy and nursing practice.* New York: McGraw-Hill Book Company, 1981.

American Academy of Nursing Task Force on Nursing Practice in Hospitals. *Magnet hospitals attraction and retention of professional nurses.* Kansas City, Mo.: American Nurses' Association, 1983.

American Nurses' Association National Task Force on Education for Nursing Practice. *Education for nursing practice in the context of the 1980s.* Kansas City, Mo.: American Nurses' Association, 1983.

Annas, G. J., Glantz, L. H. & Katz, B. F. *The rights of doctors, nurses, and allied health professionals.* New York: Avon Books, 1981.

Ashley, J. A. *Hospitals, paternalism and the role of the nurse.* New York: Teachers College, 1976.

Beauchamp, T. L. & Perlin, S. *Ethical issues in death and dying.* Englewood Cliffs, N.J.: Prentice-Hall, Inc., 1978.

Bullough, B. *The law and the expanding nursing role* (2nd ed.). New York: Appleton-Century-Crofts, 1980.

Bullough, B., Bullough, V. L. & Soukup, M.C. *Nursing issues and nursing strategies for the eighties.* New York: Springer Publishing Co., 1983.

Bullough, V. L.*The care of the sick: the emergence of modern nursing.* New York: Prodist, 1978.

Bullough, V. L. & Bullough, B. *Health care for other Americans.* New York: Appleton-Century-Crofts, 1982.

Bullough, V. L.*The subordinate sex: a history of attitudes toward women.* New York: Penguin Books, 1974.

Chaska, N. L. *The nursing profession: a time to speak.* New York: McGraw-Hill Book Company, 1983.

Chinn, P. *Advances in nursing theory development.* Rockville, Md.: Aspen Systems, 1983.

Conway, M. E. & Andruskiw, O. *Administrative theory and practice: issues in higher education in nursing.* Norwalk, Conn.: Appleton-Century-Crofts, 1983.

Corbett, J. V. *Diagnostic procedures in nursing practice.* Norwalk, Conn.: Appleton-Century-Crofts, 1983.

Creighton, H. *Law every nurse should know* (3rd Ed.). Philadelphia, Pa.: Saunders, 1975.

Davis, A. J. & Aroskar, M. A. *Ethical dilemmas and nursing practice* (2nd Ed.). Norwalk, Conn.: Appleton-Century-Crofts, 1983.

Doudera, A. E. & Peters, J. D. (Eds.). *Legal and ethical aspects of treating critically and terminally ill patients.* Ann Arbor, Mich.: AUPHA Press, 1982.

Fiesta, J. *The law & liability: a guide for nurses.* New York: John Wiley & Sons, 1983.

Folta, J. & Deck, E. *A sociological framework for patient care* (2nd Ed.). New York: John Wiley & Sons, 1979.

Fondiller, S. H. *The entry dilemma: the national league for nursing and the higher education movement, 1952–1972 with an epilogue to 1983.* New York: National League for Nursing, 1983.

Georgopoulos, B. S. (Ed.). *Organization research on health institutions.* Ann Arbor, Mich.: The Institute for Social Research, The University of Michigan, 1972.

Grissum, M. & Spengler, C. *Womanpower and health care.* Boston: Little, Brown, 1976.

Hardy, M. E. & Conway, M. E. *Role theory: Perspectives for health professionals.* New York: Appleton-Century-Crofts, 1978.

Hemelt, M. D. & Mackert, M. E. *Dynamics of law in nursing and health care.* Reston, Va.: Reston Publishing Company, 1978.

Henderson, V. *The nature of nursing.* New York: Macmillan, 1966.

Herbert, R. G. *Florence Nightingale: Saint, reformer or rebel.* Malabar, Fla., Robert E. Krieger, 1981.

Jacox, A. K. & Norris, C. M. *Organizing for independent nursing practice.* New York: Appleton-Century-Crofts, 1977.

Jones, J. H. *Bad blood: The Tuskegee syphilis experiment.* New York: The Free Press, 1981.

Kalisch, B. & Kalisch, P. *Politics of nursing.* Philadelphia, Pa.: Lippincott, 1982.

Kalisch, P. A. & Kalisch, B. J. *The advance of American nursing.* Boston: Little, Brown, 1978.

Kelly, C. *Dimensions of professional nursing* (4th Ed.). New York: Macmillan Company, 1981.

Kim, H. S. *The nature of theoretical thinking in nursing.* Norwalk, Conn.: Appleton-Century-Crofts, 1983.

Kramer, M. *Reality shock: why nurses leave nursing.* St. Louis: C. V. Mosby, 1974.

Lagemann, E. C. (Ed.). *Nursing history: new perspectives, new possibilities.* New York: Teachers College, Columbia University, 1983.

Lenburg, C. B. *Open learning and career mobility in nursing.* St. Louis: C. V. Mosby, 1975.

Lysaught, J. P. *Acting in affirmation: toward an unambiguous profession of nursing.* New York: McGraw-Hill Book Company, 1981.

Maas, M. & Jacox, A. K. *Guidelines for nurse autonomy/patient welfare.* New York: Appleton-Century-Crofts, 1977.

Mayers, M. G., Norby, R. B. & Watson, A. B. *Quality assurance for patient care: Nursing perspectives.* New York: Appleton-Century-Crofts, 1977.

Muff, J. (Ed.). *Socialization, sexism and stereotyping.* St. Louis: C. V. Mosby, 1982.

Montag, M. & Gotkin, L. C. *Community college education for nursing.* New York: McGraw-Hill Book Company, 1959.

National Commission for the Study of Nursing and Nursing Education. *An abstract for action.* New York: Blakeston, 1970.

National Commission on Nursing. *Initial report and preliminary recommendations.* Chicago: The Hospital Research and Educational Trust, 1981.

National Commission on Nursing. *Summary report and recommendations.* Chicago: The Hospital Research and Educational Trust, 1983.

National Commission for the Study of Nursing and Nursing Education, J. P. Lysaught, Director. *Action in nursing: progress in professional purpose.* New York: McGraw-Hill, 1974.

Pender, N. J. *Health promotion in nursing practice.* Norwalk, Conn.: Appleton-Century-Crofts, 1982.

Phaneuf, M. C. *The nursing audit: self-regulation in nursing practice* (2nd Ed.). New York: Appleton-Century-Crofts, 1976.

President's Commission for the Study of Ethical Problems in Medicine and Biomedical and Behavioral Research. *Making health care decisions. A report on the ethical and legal implications of informed consent in the patient-practitioner relationship, Volume one: report.* Washington, D.C.: U.S. Government Printing Office, October 1982.

Price, J. L. & Meuller, C. W. *Professional turnover: The case of nurses.* New York: S. P. Medical and Scientific Books, 1981.

Record, J. C. (Ed.). *Staffing primary care in 1990: physician replacement and cost savings.* New York: Springer Publishing Company, 1981.

Riehl, J. P. & Roy, C. (Eds.). *Conceptual models for nursing practice* (2nd Ed.). New York: Appleton-Century-Crofts, 1980.

Roemer, M. I. *Rural health care.* St. Louis: C. V. Mosby, 1976.

Russell, O. R. *Freedom to die: Moral and legal aspects of euthanasia.* New York: Human Sciences Press, 1975.

Safier, G. *Contemporary American leaders in nursing: An oral history.* New York: McGraw-Hill Book Company, 1977.

Southwick, A. F. *The law of hospital and health care administration.* Ann Arbor, Mich.: Health Administration Press, University of Michigan, 1978.

Spector, E. *Cultural diversity in health and illness.* New York: Appleton-Century-Crofts, 1979.

Styles, M. M. *On nursing: toward a new endowment.* St. Louis: C. V. Mosby Company, 1982.

Sultz, H. A., Zielezney, M., Gentry, J. M. & Kinyon, L. *Longitudinal study of nursing practitioners, phase III.* Washington, D.C.: U.S. Government Printing Office, 1980.

Summary Report of the Graduate Medical National Advisory Committee, Vols. 1–7. Washington, D.C.: U.S. Government Printing Office, HRA Publications 81-65-657, 1980.

The National Joint Practice Commission. *Together: A casebook of joint practices in primary care.* Chicago, Ill.: National Joint Practice Commission, 1977.

The Report of the Committee. *The study of credentialing in nursing: A new approach.* Kansas City, Mo.: American Nurses' Association, 1979.

U.S. Department of Health and Human Services, Public Health Service. *Prevention '82.* Washington, D.C.: DHHS (PHS) Publication No. 82-50157, 1983.

U.S. Department of Health and Human Services, Public Health Service. *Nursing practice at the bedside: Strategies for the eighties. Report of an invitational workship September 22–24, 1981.* E. P. Lewis (Ed.). Washington, D.C.: DHHS Publication No. HRS-P-DN-83-2.

Walker, L. O. & Avant, K. C. *Strategies for theory construction in nursing.* Norwalk, Conn.: Appleton-Century-Crofts, 1983.

Weeks, L. E. & Berman, H. J. (Eds.). *Economics in health care.* Germantown, Md.: Aspen Systems Corporation, 1977.

Woodham-Smith, C. *Florence Nightingale 1820–1910.* New York: McGraw-Hill Book Company, 1951.

Wooldridge, P. J., Schmitt, M. H., Skipper, J. K. & Leonard, R. C. *Behavioral science & nursing theory.* St. Louis: C. V. Mosby Company, 1983.

Yura, H. & Walsh, M. B. The nursing process: assessing, planning, implementing, evaluating (4th Ed.). Norwalk, Conn.: Appleton-Century-Crofts, 1983.

ARTICLES

Aiken, L. H., Glendon, R. J. & Rogers, D. D. The shortage of hospital nurses: A new perspective. *American Journal of Nursing,* September 1981, 1612–1618.

Aiken, L. Nursing's future: Public policies, private actions. *American Journal of Nursing,* October 1983, 83, 1440–1444.

Balint, J., Menninger, K. & Hurt, M. Job opportunities for master's prepared nurses. *Nursing Outlook,* March/April 1983, 109–114.

Bem, S. L. The measurement of psychological androgyny. *Journal of Consulting and Clinical Psychology,* 1974, 42(2), 155–162.

Bullough, B. Prescribing authority for nurses. *Nursing Economics,* September/October 1983, 1, 122–125.

Bullough, B. Legislative update: Vague umbrella nurse practice acts in trouble: The case of Missouri. *Pediatric Nursing,* March/April 1983, 9, 142.

Capuzzi, C. Power and interest groups: A study of ANA and AMA. *Nursing Outlook,* August 1980, 28, 478–482.

Davis, C. K. The federal role in changing health care financing, part I. *Nursing Economics,* July/August 1983, 10–17.

Davis, C. K. The federal role in changing health care financing, part II. *Nursing Economics,* September/October 1983, 98–104, 146.

Dayani, E. C. Professional and economic self-governance in nursing. *Nursing Economics,* July/August 1983, 20–23.

Diers, D. Nursing reclaims its role. *Nursing Outlook,* September/October 1982, 30, 459–463.

Edmunds, M. Nurse practitioner-physician competition. *Nurse Practitioner*, March/April 1981, 6, 47, 49, 53–54.

Fagin, C. Nursing as an alternative to high cost care. *American Journal of Nursing*, January 1982, 82, 56–60.

Fromer, M. J. Abortion ethics. *Nursing Outlook*, April 1982, 30, 234–240.

Goldwater, M. From a legislator: Views on third-party reimbursement for nurses. *American Journal of Nursing*, March 1982, 82, 411–414.

Gortner, S. R. Research in nursing: The federal interest and grant program. *American Journal of Nursing*, 1973, 73, 1052–1055.

Greenleaf, N. P. Labor force participation among registered nurses and women in comparable occupations. *Nursing Research*, September/October 1983, 32, 306–311.

Griffith, H. Strategies for direct third-party reimbursement for nurses. *American Journal of Nursing*, March 1982, 82, 408–411.

Jacox, A. Significant questions about IOM's study of nursing. *Nursing Outlook*, January/February 1983, 31, 28–33.

Kalisch, B. J. & Kalisch, P. A. Improving the image of nursing. *American Journal of Nursing*, January 1983, 83, 48–52.

Kramer, M. Philosophical foundations of baccalaureate nursing education. *Nursing Outlook*, April 1981, 29, 224–228.

Lynaugh, J. The entry into practice conflict: How we got where we are and what will happen next. *American Journal of Nursing*, February 1980, 266–270.

Rogers, M. Nursing: To be or not to be. *Nursing Outlook*, January 1974, 20, 42–46.

Stein, L. I. The doctor-nurse game. *Archives of General Psychiatry*, June 1967, 16, 699–703.

Sultz, H. A., Henry, O. M., Kinyon, L. J., Buck, G. M. & Bullough, B. A decade of change for nurse practitioners, Part I. *Nursing Outlook*, May/June 1983, 31, 138–141, 188.

Sultz, H. A., Henry, O. M., Kinyon, L. J., Buck, G. M. & Bullough, B. A decade of change for nurse practitioners, Part II. *Nursing Outlook*, July/August 1983, 216–219.

Sultz, H. A., Henry, O. M., Kinyon, L. J., Buck, G. M. & Bullough, B. A decade of change for nurse practitioners, Part III. *Nursing Outlook*, September/October 1983, 266–269.

The Darling case. *Journal of the American Medical Association*, November 11, 1968, 206, 1665.

The Darling case revisited. *Journal of the American Medical Association*, November 18, 1968, 206, 1875.

Trandel-Korenchuk, D. & Trandel-Korenchuk, K. Borrowed servant and captain-of-the-ship doctrines. *Nurse Practitioner*, February 1982, 7, 33–34.

Wandelt, M. Pierce, P. & Weddowson, R. Why nurses leave nursing and what can be done about it. *American Journal of Nursing*, January 1981, 81, 72–77.

Index